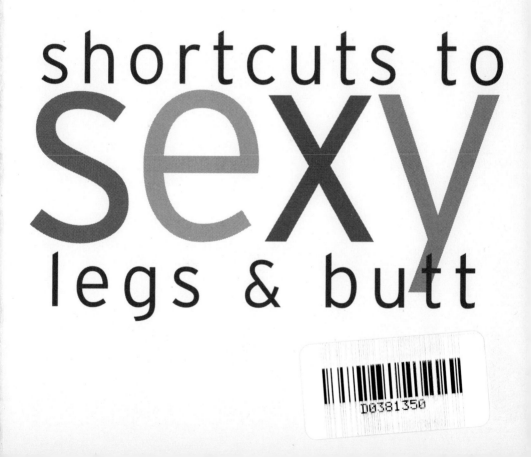

shortcuts to
sexy
legs & butt

# shortcuts to sexy
## legs & butt

### CHERYL FENTON

337 ways to trim, tone, camouflage, and beautify

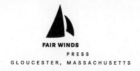

FAIR WINDS
PRESS
GLOUCESTER, MASSACHUSETTS

First published in the USA in 2004 by
Fair Winds Press
33 Commercial Street
Gloucester, MA 01930

10 9 8 7 6 5 4 3 2 1

ISBN 1-59233-085-1

Library of Congress Cataloging-in-Publication Data available


Cover and book design by Laura McFadden Design, Inc.
laura.mcfadden@rcn.com

Printed and bound in Canada

The information in this book is for educational purposes only. It is not intended to
replace the advice of a physician or medical practitioner. Please see your health care
provider before beginning any new health program.

*For my family and Samantha, who get me off my butt to always follow my dreams; for Marty, Jeff, and Whitney, who have held me up when life made my legs weak; and for Ida Natoli Raitano.*

# [contents]

# The Natoli Butt

WHY I WROTE THIS BOOK

**I was 13.** That's when it happened.

It wasn't my first crush or my first crushing heart-break. It wasn't nature telling me, "You're a woman now." It was worse. ▪ It was when it was brought to my attention that I have a bubble butt. ▪ It happened on an innocent night when my family was getting ready for a dinner out. I twirled and twirled in front of my full-length mirror like a catwalker-in-training. I made my debut at the bottom of the stairs in my newest black dress from Limited Express and asked, "How do I look?" My mother swelled with pride and answered, "Well, you certainly have the Natoli butt."

Yes, the rounded Natoli-family fanny that was birthed on an island off of Italy's southern coast had now reared its legacy all over my third generation rear. There was nowhere to run. It followed me everywhere.

Until that day, my gams and glutes weren't things I thought about much. I didn't worry about cramming my legs into the season's latest style of jeans or making them fuzz-free for a romp in the sand. Running, skipping, jumping—my legs simply took me from place to place. And my butt…well, that was what I fell on when my little sister Valerie and I would run around on a slippery floor in our fluffy socks. Try telling a girl who plays in creeks and saves puddle-stranded worms that she will someday consider a purple leg bruise a reason to wear pants, not a badge of honor.

But the day did arrive when I realized that a girl's legs could lead to something more than just the nearest tree house. How could they not? There had to be something behind Rod Stewart belting out the words to "Hot Legs" and ZZ Top warning us that "she knows how to use them." Whether I liked it or not, I was growing into a 5'8" young woman—legs, butt, and all. So, armed with leg-emphasizing stirrup pants, screams from Jane Fonda to clench my buttocks, and the most fabulous leg warmers that a misguided fashion slave of the '80s could buy, my lower half became a new project.

So began my quest to make the best out of my legs and rear end. I wanted them to be leaner, firmer. And I decided my butt can stay a bubble, just not a droopy, deflated one.

Don't get me wrong. I've never been unhappy with my size-6 frame. I've been blessed with a metabolism that hasn't let me (or my butt) down. But there is always a brief moment of panic when hemlines crawl up a bit. My eyes roll and a sigh of "here we go again" escapes me every year that minis become majors in a season's wardrobe and tight jeans become more than a casual alternative. I question, Are my legs toned enough to carry off a short BCBG skirt? How will my butt look when I shoehorn it into those low-rise Seven jeans? And, regardless of how thin, toned, and fit I am, there is always the dreaded swimsuit issue (thanks, *Sports Illustrated*). I'm convinced that a day at the beach sends even the leggiest of supermodels into a state of panic, whether they will admit it or not. (At least that's what I tell myself.)

As a beauty, health, and fitness writer, everywhere I look, from the runways of fashion shows to the glossy ads of my favorite magazines, I see lengthy legs and firm, rounded backsides. Short skirts with skyscraper-high heels waltzing down the red carpet; tight, low-rise jeans revealing just the top of a firm bottom; women shaking their perfectly rounded rears in the camera of a hip-hop music video. How can anyone ignore the leggy models and celebs that seem to appear everywhere we look?

There's no need to panic, though. I'm not about to tell you to starve yourself or to plan on exercising five times a day. Great legs and butts aren't about extreme weight loss or overdoing the workouts. Gone are the super skinny legs of the '60s Twiggies. Women are no longer teetering on sticks and sitting on bony butts. Today's legs are strong and muscular, chiseled and toned. Women are celebrating their curves and relishing the view from behind.

Now that I'm climbing (the stair stepper) into my early 30s I know that my legs do more than get me from point A to point B. They get me looks when they peek out from underneath a tiny mini. They make me feel strong as I Rollerblade up a steep hill faster than girls half my age. They bring me confidence as I stand tall during a freelance article pitch.

Not everyone can have 56-inch legs and a perfect derriere, but if you think that a jiggly bum and flabby thighs are your destiny, you are sorely mistaken. After reading the information I have gathered, say sayonara saddlebags and hello to gorgeous legs and a great rear end. ~

# [introduction]

**Unless you were born with it,** no amount of exercise will give you that perfect derriere. And unless you were born tall, no one can add length to your legs. But training your leg and butt muscles can make them leaner, tighter, and firmer, giving you more lift where you want it and less jiggle where you don't. This book will give you all the quick tips and tricks you need to get the backside and lean legs that you have always wanted.

Remember, you can't choose where you gain weight, so that means you can't choose where you lose it, either. Like hair, eyes, and recipes for chicken soup, the shapes of your butt and legs are passed down through your family. Take a look at your parents or other relatives. Genetics will decide how much your butt and legs can really change.

And being a woman doesn't help matters. We are genetically predisposed to hang on to that unwanted weight on our thighs and butts because these are the main storage areas for body fat meant to help us survive a famine. But in a country where more than two-thirds of us are considered overweight and you can't swing a Twinkle without hitting a donut, we obviously don't have to worry about where our next meal is coming from. Well, try telling that to Mother Nature. She still insists on sticking to her plan.

## Your Lower Half

The average woman has only 56 percent of the upper body strength of a man. Her lower body strength is another story. There she has a whopping

72 percent—now we're talking. It's not important for you to know every single muscle strand in your legs and butt, but it's good to have an understanding of what you are working, whether it's what you're strutting through a club on a Friday night or focusing on at the gym. The main muscles are:

- Gluteus maximus
- Biceps femoris
- Gluteus minimus
- Vastus lateralist
- Gluteus medius
- Gracilis

## 1. The gluteus maximus.

This is the largest muscle in your buttocks. Known as the upper buttocks, this outermost muscle originates on the outer edge of your pelvis and attaches to the rear thighbone. It extends your hip, lifts your leg behind you, and rotates your thighbones outward.

## 2. The vastus lateralist.

The largest quad muscle, it's the outer mass that covers the front and the side of your upper leg bone. This large muscle helps to bend your leg and extend your knee.

### 3. The biceps femoris.

These are the hamstrings—the backs of your thighs. These muscles work with the gluteus maximus during hip extension and engaged when you flex your knees.

### 4. The gluteus medius.

Your upper hip abductor is attached to your pelvis and the top of your thighbone. This muscle moves the leg out and away from the center of your body with the help of the gluteus minimus.

### 5. The gluteus minimus.

This is the outer hip abductor, located under the thighbone.

### 6. The gracilis.

These are the inner thighs, also known as the hip adductors.

## Working for Your Specific Body Type

The type of overall fitness routine you will want to follow depends
on your body type. Do you have the plump, heart-shaped butt of a
voluptuous body or the smaller, more muscular behind of a boyish
figure? To find out where your legs and butt stand, take this test. Put
your hand around your wrist. If your thumb and middle finger overlap,
you are an ectomorph; if they touch, you are a mesomorph; if they do
not touch at all, you are an endomorph.

• **Ectomorphic:** You are thin and have difficulty gaining weight. If you
want to build a more rounded butt and more shapely legs, spend time
in the weight room. Think about a squat or two to build more muscle
mass.

• **Mesomorphic:** You are naturally muscular, well-formed, and athletic.
You have more fast-twitch muscles (these are the muscles that give you
power). Your butt and legs can get muscular, but don't plan on them
ever being petite.

• **Endomorphic:** You have a round or pear-shaped body. If you want a smaller butt and thinner hips and legs, forget about spot training in the beginning. This will only make your gluteus more maximus. Concentrate on overall weight loss through dieting and fat-burning activities like cycling, jogging, and kickboxing.

Here are a few other tips to consider when you're working toward your ultimate weight-loss goals.

• If you are trying to build muscle, three to five 20- to 30-minute cardio workouts per week is the way to go. Most of your workout should be moderate to high intensity.

• If you are trying to maintain your weight, three to five 20- to 45-minute moderate cardio workouts a week should cover your needs.

• If you are trying to lose weight, try doing five or six 30- to 60-minute cardio workouts a week. Twice a week, increase your intensity to burn extra calories, boost your metabolism, and build muscle.

Strength training goes hand-in-hand with cardio. Using weights is the perfect way to work each muscle group to complete your routine. When choosing weights to help take your own weight off, don't overdo it. The perfect amount of weight should leave you struggling during the last two reps of the set, not struggling from the beginning.

Many women avoid weights because they think they'll bulk up. In reality, though, very few women have the capacity to build huge muscles because they don't have enough testosterone in their body. If you are exercising and it still seems that your rear is expanding faster than you want, don't stop weight training. It may be that you aren't losing body fat even though you're building muscle. Turn to nutrition to lose the fat.

A successful toning and strengthening workout doesn't always need to involve a lot of movement. With static movements and stretches, yoga and Pilates are great ways to quietly work your legs and butt, not to mention calm your mind and spirit.

## Using This Book

Reading this book from start to finish is certainly a great first step toward a better bottom half. But to help you make the big world of weight loss a little smaller, I've created specific sections for when you have an event for which you want to look your best—the big date, a fantastic party, weekends at play, the 9-to-5 grind, or a beach day. Using my tips on beauty, fitness, nutrition, and fashion, you will be able to improve your legs and rear view.

This book offers suggestions on preparing yourself for your plans, from weeks in advance to during the big event. These tips will help you do everything you can to ensure that you will have the can't-stop-looking-at-them legs and pinchable butt you've always wanted. The Health and Beauty Bytes sections will teach you ways to take care of the skin you're in, and the Fashion Facts portions will help you cover (or uncover) it all with leg- and butt-flattering fashion. Rely on Fitness Fun for exercise tips to help you target those specific areas that need firming, and look to Nutrition Nuggets for the right fuel to maintain your trim and toned gams.

As you perform these shortcuts and quick fixes, there is one thing to remember: At the end of the day, it takes a healthy diet and an exercise program to maintain good health and overall strength for your entire body, not just your legs and butt. If you faithfully follow the longer-term fitness programs I've prepared, you will see noticeable differences in the firmness of your legs and butt within 4 to 6 weeks. Almost everyone sees a big difference within 10 weeks.

So get ready to create that fine physique you've wanted for so long. It's time to put your best foot forward and continue that stride with a pair of shapely legs and a firm bottom. ~

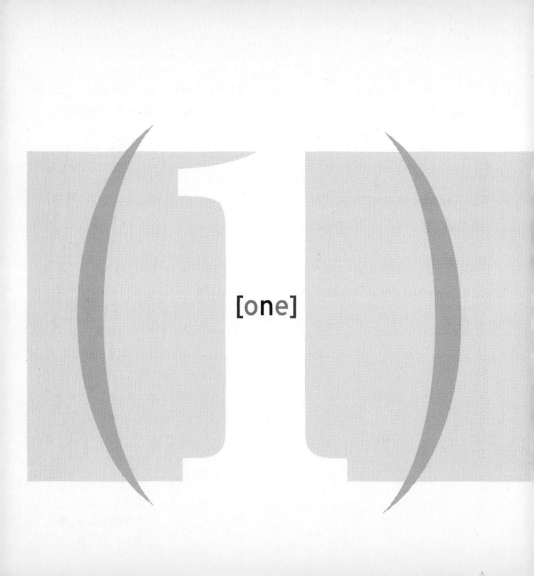

[one]

# The Big Date

**It may be with your husband,** your husband-to-be, or a man bordering on Mr. Right. Or maybe it's just that all-important first impression you're going for. Whatever the date, there will come a time when you want to impress a man in your life with your shapely stems and your sculpted butt. After all, your mind and heart are already beautiful on their own. But your body might need a little boost.

This chapter will help you exercise for the firmest derriere, offer beauty tips on creating touchable legs, and give you hints on finding outfits that will guarantee dates two, three, four, five, and beyond. With the right plan in place, he'll be dropping his napkin during dinner just to catch glimpses of your fantastic lower half. And somewhere between the low-fat grilled salmon and the not-so-low-fat crème brûlée, he'll fall in love for the first time (or all over again). ~

Health and Beauty Bytes

## (1) Mask your "flaws"

Before you clean up, get dirty! Do as the French do and cover your legs and cheeks in a mud mask to draw out toxins from your skin. Mud masks are available at drugstores for just a few dollars and even though they say they're for your face, feel free to slather them on your legs and butt! Then shower the mud away to reveal great skin underneath.

## (2) A firming lotion

Firming lotions help you to achieve a more toned look. The key ingredients (such as copper, Co-enzyme Q10, Biotin, and caffeine) help to repair the skin's elasticity, which naturally decreases with age. Smooth on your legs and butt twice a day to help repair the skin's collagen and make it look younger and more toned.

## (3) Moisturize more than once daily

Who says that moisturizer should only be applied in the morning? Multiple applications of moisturizer throughout the day will keep your legs silky smooth and help you avoid out-of-control dry skin. Tuck a travel-size lotion into your purse and duck into the bathroom for a mid-date moisturize. And don't overlook the inexpensive products. They may not have pretty packaging or exotic scents, but products like Vaseline, Aquaphor, and Eucerin provide inexpensive relief for rough skin.

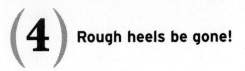

## **(4)** Rough heels be gone!

Make sure your toes are presentable—not only for open-toe strappy sandals, but also for any spur-of-the-moment foot rubs. The night before your date, soak your feet for 10 minutes in lukewarm water, rubbing your heels afterward with a pumice stone. Massage in rich creams with peppermint oils and cover up with a pair of thick cotton socks. In the morning, wake to touchable tootsies.

## **(5)** You can "scents" his attraction

Dab a little perfume on your ankles. Like heat, fragrance rises. To cover more leg area, dust on the powder version of a perfume. Let your mood for the night pick the fragrance.

- **Romantic:** Sweet-smelling flowers, including rose, freesia, and lilac.
- **Exotic:** Light notes with spicy oriental essences like lotus flowers.

- **Flirty:** Citrus scents, green smells like freshly cut stems, crisp florals (mandarin flower, hyacinth) with musk, spice, or sandalwood.
- **Sexy:** Spicy flowers (ylang-ylang, jasmine, or narcissus) or lush fruits (plums or black currants) with something warm or musky (spice, amber, or patchouli).
- **Cozy:** Comfort food scents like vanilla, ginger, or almond.

# ( 6 ) Lighten up!

Perfume a little heavier than you intended? It's a fixable faux pas. Blot the offending spot with a cotton ball dampened with rubbing alcohol, a trick used by perfumers to lighten fragrances during production.

# ⑦ Sweets for the sweet

Sweeten the deal for your date with a sugar body scrub. The sweet stuff has great exfoliating properties, while the oils add softness to your delicious derriere and legs. Removing dead skin from your legs will leave them touchable and soft, with a certain shine. Buff in a circular motion, starting from the ankles up, and rinse with warm water. The company Fresh makes a great brown sugar body polish, or try this at-home recipe:

## Brown Sugar Body Buff

- ½ cup brown sugar
- ½ cup fine sea salt
- ¼ cup of a combination of sunflower, sweet almond, and jojoba oils
- 1 tablespoon kaolin
- 1 tablespoon honey
- 1 teaspoon vitamin E oil
- 1 teaspoon each of three of your favorite essential oils

Mix the ingredients together in a small bowl. Stir before use. Makes 8 ounces.

## ( 8 ) Get milk

Pour a cup or more of powdered milk under running bath water and step into luxury. The lactic acid in the milk will remove dry, dead skin and leave your legs baby soft. Milk protein also forms a film on the skin that allows it to retain moisture, plus it gives skin a glossy finish and fine touch. Just add a drop or two of some scented oil if you want a really dreamy bath.

## ( 9 ) Bring his eye elsewhere

If you are feeling self-conscious about your butt or legs, make sure that his eyes are focused above your problem areas. This means accessories. Try draping a brilliant scarf around your long, thin neck.

# (**10**) Shaving secrets

You might bounce out of bed the morning of the Big Date, ready to grab your razor. Not so fast! Follow this shaving advice and you'll have the smoothest gams possible—with the least amount of pain and suffering.

- **Don't shave when you first wake up.** Body fluids make skin puffy and more difficult to shave. Wait 20 to 30 minutes.

- **Do wet hair first for at least 3 minutes.** Plumped, hydrated skin forces hair to stand up.

- **Do lightly exfoliate with a washcloth.** This will remove dead skin that might impede the razor. But don't rub away too much, or razor burn might be in your future.

- **Don't shave after being in a bath for too long.** After 8 minutes the skin shrivels, making it harder to get a close shave.

- **Don't use a dull razor.** Dull blades cause more nicks than new ones do, and they also increase your chances of ingrown hairs.

- **Do allow shaving cream or gel to sit on the skin for 2 minutes.** It helps moisturize the skin and keep hair erect.

# (11) Accept compliments

Chances are, you'll look so great after following the advice here that you'll be getting a "Wow!" or a glazed look of speechless adoration. So learn how to take a compliment. It shows confidence, not vanity. Don't bat the kind words away…they are a gift. And after all, you deserve them. Return compliments with a simple smile and a "thank you."

*Fitness Fun*

# (12) Get a rubdown

Besides the obvious oooohs and aaaahs of delight, massage can actually enhance your skin's condition and get rid of cellulite temporarily, smoothing the appearance of your legs and butt. Massage directly improves the function of the oil and sweat glands, which keep the skin lubricated, clean, and cooled. Rough and tough skin can become softer and suppler. Try a Swedish massage for the beginner or a deep tissue massage for the brave. For even more serious cellulite reduction, try Endermologie—a massage system that uses a double-headed rolling and suction action.

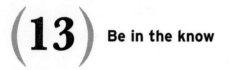 **Be in the know**

When getting a massage:

- Ask if the masseuse is licensed. Currently 33 states have passed laws that regulate massage therapy. Ask if the masseuse is a member of the American Massage Therapy Association.
- Remove your clothing only to your level of comfort. It's not unusual to be au naturel, so don't feel inhibited.
- Be honest. Give background information, such as medical history, stress levels, and any painful areas. And if the masseuse hits a spot during the massage that you don't enjoy or that you want them to focus more on, speak up!

# (14) Sassy salsa

Sway those hips and move those arms like a Latin lovely for sexy legs.
Stand with your feet together. Step your right foot forward for one
count, then back with a cha, cha, cha. Then it's your left foot's turn to
go back and then to the center for one step. Cha, cha, cha! To shake it
up, step to the right side with your right foot, then back. Then step to
the left with your left foot for one count, then back. This sexy, steamy
dance burns around 125 calories per hour.

# (15) Standing leg lifts

Make a stand for great thigh muscles and toned hip flexors! Stand with
your back and the palms of your hands against a wall. Spread your
feet several inches apart. Exhale and gently raise your right leg as high as
you can. Hold. Inhale and slowly lower your leg. Lift forward eight times.
Then lift to the side eight times. Switch legs and repeat. Do two sets.

# (16) Squat raises

Instead of plain old squats, Jennifer Lopez (and her famous behind) love these "squat raises" to tone up her lower half: With feet shoulder-width apart, bend your knees slightly and lower your body until you're almost sitting. Rise back up and onto your toes. Do two sets of 25. (For even more butt-whooping work, jump up out of the squat.)

# (17) Easy does it

Exercise, much like romance, is best when done slowly, so don't rush through your workout routine. You'll get more of a challenge if your movements are slow and controlled. Isolate each muscle that you are working and really think about what you're doing. Slow and steady.

# (18)) Lunge with cross chop

Sweep away fat before you sweep your date off his feet! With your feet hip-width apart, hold a broom in both hands in front of you. Raise your left knee to hip level and raise your arms overhead. Take a long step back with your left foot and lower your left knee to the floor. At the same time, draw the broom down and across the front of your body. Pause, and return to standing. Repeat 10 to 12 times, then switch legs.

# (19)) If you can make it here...

Stand tall and hold your arms straight out to your sides. Kick your right leg out Rockette-style, then your left. Swivel at the waist with each kick to work your abs, too. Do this to exhaustion (or until the house lights come up).

# ( **20** ) Skate—inline or on ice

Whether it's a winter wonderland or a lovely summer day, throw on a pair of skates. The sweeping movement works your legs and butt, targeting the pesky saddlebag areas. So blade down the path or take a loop around a local ice rink. A 130-pound woman burns between 320 and 400 calories per hour.

# ( **21** ) The chair

Stand with your back against a wall. Slide down until your thighs are parallel to the floor. Hold for up to three minutes. The perfect move to do while waiting for your date to arrive.

## Be a prima ballerina

If you're going to drag him to the ballet, you might as well get in the mood—minus the tutu, of course. Former dancer Florence Tambone recommends these willowy movements to tone and stretch your legs and butt. During these exercises, keep your carriage (torso) lifted, your abs strong, your glutes tight, and your shoulders down. Warm up for five minutes with a weight-bearing exercise like jogging in place.

# (22) Stretching

Place a leg up in front of you on a counter or table no higher than is comfortable. Feel the stretch in the hamstring as you slowly fall forward and bring your arms toward your foot. Hold for 20 seconds. With your leg still up, turn and face the side, as you fall down to reach toward your standing leg. Hold for 20 seconds, then switch legs.

## $\left(23\right)$ Plié (1st position)

One of the most basic ballet movements is designed to improve posture and strengthen and tone legs without creating bulk. Turn your feet out and keep your heels together. Keep your knees over your toes and your back straight. Lower as far as you can go until you feel the stretch in your calves; then lift up on your toes and continue down as far as you can. Come back up slowly, squeezing your inner thighs together. Perform four sets of 15 reps.

## $\left(24\right)$ Plié (2nd position)

Place your feet farther than shoulder-width apart. Turn your feet out, keeping your knees over your toes. Lower down until your thighs are parallel to the floor, then lift up on your toes, then lower onto flat feet. Raise up and down on your toes 15 times. Slowly raise back up to starting position. Do four sets.

## $\left(25\right)$ Brushing leg lifts

Stand with a chair or a countertop to your right side. Place your hand a bit in front of you for stability. Keep your arm steady and your elbow bent. Push out with your left toe, dragging it along the floor, until your leg is straight in front of you. Return to start. Repeat the motion to the side. Return to start, then to the back. Do three sets of 10 before turning so the counter is on your left. Repeat with your right leg.

## $\left(26\right)$ Straight leg lifts

Standing in the same position as for Brushing Leg Lifts, straighten your leg with your toe pointed out. Brush it forward, but add a kick up. Repeat the motion to the back without falling forward. Do three sets of 10 before turning to work your right leg.

# (27) Meditate

What am I going to wear? What's my hair doing? Will we make our 7:30 pm reservation? All these little stresses can not only plague the all-important evening, but they can also wreak havoc on your hips. Stress can cause weight gain. To combat worries, try meditation. This simple practice will add a little relaxation to your evening's plans. To begin, sit in a comfortable position with your hands on your lap and your fingers open, not touching. Close your eyes. Take in the sounds around you. Notice your breath going in and out. Bring awareness to your fingers. Wiggle them slightly and feel the warmth in them. Bring your thumb and index finger together on each hand and draw your awareness to the point above and between your eyebrows, known as your third eye. Try to feel a sense of warmth there. Now bring a peaceful and pleasant image into your mind, such as a beach or mountain. Keep your focus on the third eye and your image for about five minutes. When you feel ready, open your eyes.

# workbook

## A longer, leaner you

Strengthen and stretch to make your leg muscles longer and leaner.

## $(28)$ Couch cobra

Strengthens arms, abs, quads; stretches chest, back, hip flexors, hamstrings, quads. Lie facedown on the edge of a couch or bed, positioning your left foot on the floor, aligned with your shoulder, and extending your right leg behind you on the couch or bed. Lift your chest and steady yourself with your hands in front. Bend your right leg and reach behind with your right hand to grasp your right ankle. Lower your right leg to the start. Switch legs and repeat. Do 5 to 10 reps on each side.

## $\left(29\right)$ T stand

Strengthens abs, back, hamstrings; stretches inner thighs, hip flexors, hamstrings. Stand with your feet together. Slowly bend from your hips to lower your torso, touching your fingers to the floor. Lift your right leg behind you to hip height, keeping hips level. Hold for five counts. Return to start and repeat on the other side. Do 5 to 10 reps on each side.

## $\left(30\right)$ Leg lift

Strengthens abs, hips, quads; stretches hamstrings, outer thighs. Sit on the edge of a sturdy chair, feet flat on the floor. Holding the sides of the chair, lift your legs to hip level. Press your feet together. Hold, then lower to start. Do three sets of 5 to 10 reps.

# (31) Have a ball!

Use a balance ball to work your leg and hip muscles for a well-rounded stretching routine. Gaiam (www.gaiam.com) has several options for balls, along with videos, DVDs, and resistance cables to use with the ball. Here are a few stretches they suggest:

- Sit on the ball and stretch one leg in front of you, in the air. Grasp that leg at the calf, hold for 15 counts, then use both hands to guide the leg down again to the ground. Repeat with the other leg.

- Sit on the ball close to a wall, put one hand on the wall for balance, and place the opposite ankle onto your knee, opening the hip. Let that knee drop toward the ground and then sit up tall and hinge forward at the hips about an inch or two. Feel the stretch in the butt and outer thigh.

- Lay face up on top of the ball. Stretch your legs and arms far away from you, as you feel a stretch in your back. Roll around to feel what other stretches your body is craving.

## Leg and butt weight machines

Those intimidating machines at the gym are actually some of the best ways to target the muscles in your legs and butt. Don't use too much weight; you should struggle a little with only the last rep of each set. Do two or three sets of 10 to 12 reps with each machine, depending on your strength level.

## (32) Standing calf-raise (works calves)

Stand tall with your heels hanging off the edge of the foot platform and shoulders under the padded weight bar. Keep your back straight, abs pulled in, and knees locked. Rise up on your tiptoes as high as you can go. Hold for a moment and lower your heels back down, past the starting place to dip below the platform. Feel a good stretch throughout the length of your calves. Hold for a moment before moving into the next rep.

# ( 33 ) Leg press (works butt and thighs)

Place your feet hip-width apart with your toes pointed forward and your heels directly behind your toes. Pull your abs in and rest your head on the back pad. Pressing through your heels, push against the platform until your legs are straight, being careful not to lock them. Bend your knees until your thighs are parallel with the platform.

# ( 34 ) Leg extension (works quads)

Bend your knees and swing your legs around so that the tops of your shins are resting against the undersides of the ankle pads. Sit up tall and pull in your abs. Straighten your legs to lift the ankle bar until your knees are straight. Hold for a second at the top position, and then slowly bend your legs back to the starting position.

## $\left(35\right)$ Leg curl (works hamstrings)

Lie down, rest your forearms on the support pad, and grasp the handles.

Gently flex your feet. Pull your abs in and turn your hips down so that your

hip bones press into the pad. Bend your knees to lift the ankle bar until

your calves are perpendicular to the floor. Slowly straighten your legs.

## $\left(36\right)$ Adductors (works inner thighs)

Sit up tall and press your knees inward until you feel tension in your

inner thighs. Hold the position for a moment, and then slowly allow your

legs to move apart.

# $(37)$ Abductors (works outer thighs)

Press your knees outward until you feel tension in your outer thighs and
the sides of your hips. Hold the position for a moment, then slowly allow
your legs to move inward again. Proper form is everything, but change
is good. You will want to perform controlled repetitions and keep your
hips stationary. But small changes in position can hit your butt and leg
muscles in different ways. Try turning out your toes or rotating your
knees out from your hips. And squeeze that butt! Contracting your glute
muscles creates even more resistance.

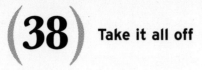

## Take it all off

Chosen a great outfit for the night? Before putting it on, take it all off! Not only does it make you feel sexy, but stripping can be a great leg and butt workout. It's great for balance, and the exercises are sensual and demanding. Combining yoga, dance, and erotic movements, this hot fitness trend has even found its way into health clubs, poles and all. If your gym doesn't offer classes, put on your sexiest push-up, some sultry music, and make up your own routine (before or after he comes to pick you up). Slowly swivel your hips, doing a few deep squat dips and slow pelvic thrusts.

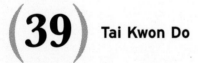

## Tai Kwon Do

High leg movements, coupled with crouching stances, give you a kick-ass leg and butt workout. Check with gyms and martial arts centers for class schedules. You can say sayonara to 380 calories per hour.

# (40) Kickboxing

It's got everything—boxing, martial arts, aerobics, kicking, and punching weighted targets. Sculpt your thighs and glutes, get out a few frustrations, and burn 350 to 450 calories per hour. Combine and alternate these moves.

- **Base move:** Quickly shift weight from the ball of one foot to the other.
- **Bob and weave:** Shift your weight back and forth while raising and lowering your torso from near-standing to near squatting. All the while, keep your elbows bent and your fisted hands in front of your face.
- **Front kick:** Kick your foot straight out in front of you with your toe up.
- **Roundhouse kick:** Swing your foot and leg up and kick so that your shoelaces hit the side of the target in front of you.
- **Side kick:** Kick with your lower torso turned inward so that your heel lands on the target while your foot is parallel to the floor.

- **Upper cut:** Start this biceps-powered punch with your fist low and end with your fist straight up.
- **Jab:** Perform quick punches at face level.
- **Hook:** Swing your fist around from the side in toward the center.

# (41) 10-minute yoga

No time for an hour-long spirit-cleansing yoga routine? Try this 10-minute practice that will clear your mind and work your legs and glutes. Each pose should be held for five deep breaths. Do both sides twice, with a 15- to 30-second pause between each rep.

- **Minute 0-2:30—Side Plank** Begin on your hands and toes in plank position (a straight-armed, straight-legged position like a push-up pose). Turn your heels to the left, resting on the outside edge of your left foot, and extend your right arm toward the ceiling. Gaze upward at your right hand and maintain a straight line from shoulders to heels.

- **Minute 2:30-5:00—Crescent Pose** Begin on your hands and toes, body in an inverted V (downward dog). Step your right foot between your hands and align your knee over your ankle. Straighten your left leg and lift your arms overhead. Press your left heel back while lifting your torso tall. Hold for five breaths, then return to downward dog.
- **Minute 5:00-7:30—Eagle Pose** Inhale, sweeping your arms high. Exhale and wrap your left arm under your right, so your elbows are at shoulder height. Press your palms together, fingers pointing up. Bend your knees 45 degrees and cross your left thigh over your right. If you can, hook your left foot around your right ankle.
- **Minute 7:30-10:00—Chair Pose** Stand with your feet parallel and hip-width apart. Inhale and raise your arms overhead, palms facing inward. Exhale and squat back as if sitting, keeping your weight over your heels as your chest moves forward. Repeat five times.

## ( **42** ) Oysters are on the menu

Order a dozen raw oysters. Not only are they an aphrodisiac, they are also rich in Vitamin A, a vitamin essential for the maintenance and healing of epithelial tissues. And with your skin being your largest expanse of epithelial tissue, this is a tasty way to make your skin more touchable.

## ( **43** ) Fork it

Keep it proper and go for foods that need to be eaten with a fork. These items will take more time to eat, leaving you more time to realize that you're full. Finger foods and quick picks also tend to be fried.

## ( **44** ) Vampires have the right idea

Garlic is a no-no, especially for the day or two before your big romantic event. Not only does it linger on your breath, but close encounters could be spoiled by the smell coming through your pores (even the pores of your legs!).

## ( **45** ) PMS=Push (away) monthly snacks

Studies show that you might consume 300 extra calories a day the week before your period. It's the carbs and sugars you crave, so try a glass of skim milk mixed with fat-free chocolate sauce. Two birds, one stone: The chocolate will solve your craving, and calcium has been found to decrease PMS symptoms.

# (46) Size matters

When following a meal plan, it's important to know a little about serving sizes. A three-ounce serving of meat, fish, or poultry is about the size of a deck of cards, and one-half cup of pasta, rice, or potatoes is about the size of a tennis ball. Here's a guide for daily serving sizes according to the Food Pyramid supplied by the U.S. Department of Agriculture and the U.S. Department of Health and Human Services.

---

**Grains:** 6 to 11 servings

• 1 slice of bread

• ½ cup cooked rice or pasta

• ½ cup of cooked cereal

• 1 ounce of ready-to-eat cereal

---

**Fruits:** 2 to 4 servings

1 medium apple, banana, or orange

---

- ¾ cup fruit juice

- ½ cup of chopped, cooked, or canned fruit

**Vegetables:** 3 to 5 servings

- ½ cup vegetables (chopped, raw, or cooked)

- 1 cup leafy raw vegetables

- ¾ cup vegetable juice

**Milk, yogurt, and cheese:** 2 to 3 servings

- 1 cup milk or yogurt

- 1½ ounces of natural cheese

- 2 ounces of processed cheese

**Meat, poultry, fish, dried beans, eggs, and nuts:** 2 to 3 servings

- ½ cup cooked beans, 1 egg, or 2 tablespoons of peanut butter

- 2 to 3 ounces of cooked lean meat, poultry, or fish

# (47) Have a cup of green tea

Not only is it teeming with disease-fighting compounds, but it also serves as a great appetite suppressant—perfect to help you get a leg up on weight loss. And if you're worried about caffeine, don't be. Green tea actually has almost less than half of the caffeine in black tea.

# (48) Get your thyroid checked

If your scale won't budge and you're actually gaining weight, or if you are losing rapidly, your thyroid may not be working well (hypothyroidism) or working too much (hyperthyroidism). That means your metabolism and fat-burning rate might be compromised. Check with your doctor. At least 13 million people suffer from hypothyroidism. In the meantime, perform this quick thyroid self-check:

1. Hold a mirror so that you can see the area of your neck just below your Adam's apple and right above your collarbone.
2. Tip your head back, while keeping this view of your neck and thyroid area in your mirror. Take a drink of water and swallow.
3. As you swallow, look at your neck. Watch carefully for any bulges, enlargement, or protrusions in this area.
4. Repeat this process several times. If you see anything that appears unusual, see your doctor right away. You may have an enlarged thyroid or a thyroid nodule, and your thyroid should be evaluated.

## (49) Watch your pounds and ounces

If you're cooking a romantic dinner at home, weigh your food as you prepare the meal to get yourself used to eating the right-size portions. Studies show that most people underestimate how much food they're eating by one-third. Putting less on your plate can mean less on your hips. And remember, ingredients are just that: ingredients. Not snacks while cooking.

# (**50**) Meds and weight gain

In a recent study, nearly 50 percent of women were wrong in thinking that their birth control pill caused weight gain. But some drugs do cause a few added pounds. Ask your doctor if you can take meds that don't have this side effect. Here are few that may cause weight gain:

1. **Birth control shot** (Depo-Provera)
2. **Mood stabilizers** (including Lithium and some epilepsy drugs)
3. **Steroids** (for asthma, lupus, or arthritis)
4. **Anti-depressants** (including Paxil, Elavil, Tofranil, Remeron, and Nardil)
5. **Meds for type 2 diabetes** (including Avandia, Actos, Diabinese, and Glucotrol)

# (51) International lean cuisine

Eating out doesn't have to mean a diet deal broken. You have plenty of tasty choices when trying delicacies from overseas.

- **Italian**—Try grilled calamari, minestrone soup, grilled fish with lemon and capers, or pizza with a little cheese and a lot of veggies.
- **Mexican**—Opt for black bean soup, fajitas, or a burrito with grilled chicken, shrimp, beans, and veggies (hold the cheese and sour cream).
- **Chinese**—Order shrimp or chicken in garlic sauce and mix it with a side order of steamed vegetables rather than rice cooked with the meal, which makes a more fattening sauce.

## (52) Olive oil vs. butter

Eaters who dipped bread in olive oil soaked up 26 percent more fat per slice than those who used butter, yet consumed less bread and fewer calories overall, according to a report in the *International Journal of Obesity*. Although olive oil contains a healthier fat than butter does, you should still take it easy on the dipping.

## (53) Slow it down

Savor the flavors and textures of your food. It takes 20 minutes for your brain to get the message from your stomach that you're full, so try to stretch the meal over at least half an hour. Take a few bites, put your fork down, and stop for a minute or two before eating again. Pay attention to your hunger symptoms, and as soon as they begin to disappear, back away from the table.

## ( 54 ) Keep it all in proportion

There is more than an ounce of truth in portions playing a part in our weight gain. Enter the French Paradox. Francophiles say *oui* to just about every no-no food out there—highly caloric sauces, rich cheeses, and decadent desserts. So how is it that only 8 percent of France's population is overweight? Their portions are $\frac{1}{3}$ to $\frac{1}{4}$ the size of ours. Don't feel it necessary to be a member of the Clean Plate Club. Take half of your meal home.

## ( 55 ) Have a glass of water before dinner

Drink a cup or two of water before you order your meal. It will fill you up and contribute to the 64 ounces a day you need for glowing skin and proper body functioning.

# (56) Don't be neurotic

Nobody likes the female cliché of constantly asking, "Does my butt look fat in these pants?" Nothing turns off a man more than a sexy women who doesn't have the confidence to wear anything but a pair of baggy sweatpants. If you don't feel comfortable wearing an outfit, change until you find something you won't fidget in.

# (57) Swing, baby, swing

Flirty swing skirts can minimize bigger behinds because they flow on and around your figure. Perfect for a dancing date, pick a skirt in flowing fabric (a silk or a sheer rayon) that has a little kick when you walk. The movement of the twirly hems will make your legs look thin and fit.

# (58) Start with what's underneath

Your underwear is as important as your outfit when it comes to looking slim. These guidelines will help you choose undergarments that won't interfere with your overall look.

- **A thong** will help you avoid bunching-up lines under your clothes that will make you look more bulky.
- **Body-shaping underwear** pulls in your hips, bottom, and tummy. A control panel in the top front of panties holds your lower stomach in.
- **Briefs or hot pants** are like small shorts, coming up to just under your belly button and covering most of your butt. These make hips look slimmer and can pull in your tummy.
- **Underwear** that cuts diagonally across the buttock lifts your bottom.
- **High-cut legs** make your legs look longer.

## (59) Love being a girl

To show off thin calves, try a below-the-knee skirt paired with a fitted sweater. This skirt length really showcases great ankles and calf muscles and adds a touch of classic femininity.

## (60) Use belts to create thinner hips

Avoid big belts, which can cut you in half visually. But tiny ones aren't the way to go, either. To create a slimmed-down look, pair a long shirt with three or four thinner belts around your hips.

## (61) Necklaces can create length

A necklace will produce a visual vertical line while drawing attention away from your lower half. Try long dangling chains or pendants, and avoid chokers. A long glamorous set of opera pearls will create the illusion of length.

## (62) Think shimmery cleavage

Distract from your derriere by bringing his attention from your lower half to your upper. Wear a low-cut wrap shirt (which slims the waistline and boosts the bust) or a little off-the-shoulder number, and add a sexy sheen to your neck, shoulders, and cleavage with shimmery lotion.

## (63) Long straight cuts=long straight figure

If you have a larger figure, pair tunics with straight-leg pants to give the appearance of an elongated figure. Tunics are also great for hiding a butt that doesn't want to be seen.

## (64) Balance it all

There is such a thing as too much of a good thing, especially when it comes to showing off a little skin. Pick one area or the other when choosing where you want to show it off. If you're wearing a short skirt, cover up on top; if you have on a low-cut blouse, don't show much leg.

## (65) Fishnet fancies

Hollywood is embracing fishnets, along with back-seamed nets that do wonders for the legs. Try colors such as nude, cocoa, and off-white to update your look. Pair fishnets with textured pants or a long, feminine skirt with a high slit for a Hollywood glam look.

## (66) Try a monochromatic look

If you wear all one color, you create the illusion of being long and thin. Only use neutral colors, like navy, brown, gray, camel, or black. But monochromatic doesn't have to mean boring. Mix textures to keep the look interesting (for example, knits with leather), or add a splash of color with a scarf tied loosely with long, dangling ends.

## (67) Know your hose

Experiment with stockings—from flirty fishnets to opaques in a range of colors. For a funkier look, wear sheer hosiery with interesting patterned graphics and textures. Stay away from horizontal lines and stripes. Not since the '60s, when miniskirts and hot pants ushered in a decade of colored and printed socks and stockings, have legs enjoyed so much exposure.

## ( **68** ) Darker colors mean a slimmer silhouette

Dark colors have a slimming effect because they absorb light rays, while lighter and brighter colors reflect them. When light is reflected, the eye has more to absorb, giving the perception of a greater space. So wear dark on your lower half to minimize a larger butt and thighs. If you have a small chest and full hips, wear a bright top and a dark bottom.

## ( **69** ) These boots are made for walking

The right height and heel on a boot can make or break an outfit. Stay away from ankle boots if you have heavier legs; instead, go for tall boots. If you like your thighs but not your calves, choose a boot up to your knee. To show off sculpted calves, try a half boot. And if you want to hide it all, try an over-the-knee boot with a skirt that comes to the top of the boot. For rounder legs, avoid stiletto heels and pointy toes; in this case, opposites are not attractive.

# (70) A little sexy lingerie

If the date goes where you hope it might, there's nothing like sexy lingerie. To make mention of your unmentionables, follow these simple guidelines:

- **Tempt him with a teddy,** which is very slimming to most figures.
- **If you're hip conscious,** wear baby doll pjs. They flare at the bottom to conceal that area.
- **A chemise nightgown** should fall just above the knees and will bring attention to great legs, while hiding problem thighs.
- **Full-length gowns** offer elegance that hides your lower half. Choose styles with sexy slits for extra taunting.
- **Tap pants** and camisole sets flare out at the thighs, making legs look thinner, while accentuating the waistline.

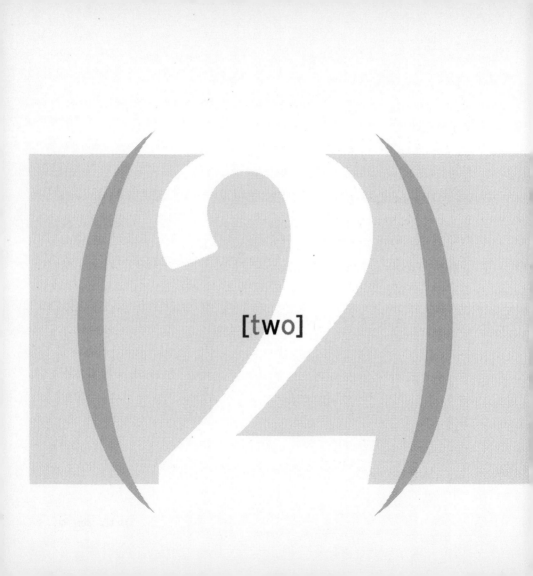

(2)

[two]

# Weekend Play

**Weekends are all about jeans.** Nothing looks better than a great-shaped butt in a perfect pair of Levis or Diesels. And when the temperatures rise, so do the hems, with your legs walking tall in short-shorts or perky peddle-pushers. But the question is, can your legs support you in style from errands to casual cocktails, whatever the season? Whether your next two days are full of grocery shopping or being the belle of the barbecue, follow this chapter to figure out how to be a jean genie out of the house and keep the doldrums (and doughnuts) away from a relaxing weekend at home. ~

# (71) Soothe tired legs

Running around a lot this weekend? To soothe aching leg muscles, add five drops each of the following extracts to steamy water and soak: eucalyptus and birch (to ease tightness), marjoram (to improve circulation), rosemary (to stimulate), and lavender (to calm).

# (72) Pimples be gone

Blemishes on your butt are a bummer. Dead skin buildup can cause red bumps on the backs of your legs and sometimes on your cheeks. Use body lotions with alpha- and beta-hydroxy acids to get rid of the culprit and speed cell turnover. Apply daily for about two weeks.

# (73) Rub like an Egyptian

Egyptian women have used crushed almonds to exfoliate their bodies for centuries. So go nuts with this at-home body mask to give an unparalleled glow to your thighs.

## Almond Mask

- 1 handful finely crushed almonds
- 5 tablespoons uncooked oatmeal
- 2 teaspoons brown sugar
- 2 tablespoons honey
- $\frac{1}{4}$ cup hot water

Mix to form a paste. Slather on and leave for 10 minutes. Massage in and rinse off.

## (74) Switch to a cream from a lotion

You should rethink your product bases during the colder months, especially if your skin is constantly dry and flaky. Creams provide a heavier hydrating base and barrier to keep moisture in and the environment out, so slather them on when temperatures drop.

## (75) Ingrown hair relief

Shaving can cause nasty bumps on your legs and bikini line that can be irritated by jeans and weekend horseplay. Soothe ingrown hairs on your calves and the backs of your thighs with salicylic-acid based products.

## ( **76** ) Humidify for hydrated skin

When temps drop and the thermostat gets turned up, humidify your environment. Your dry, itchy legs will thank you for it. Try using a portable humidifier, or simply place a pan of water on the top of your heater during cold winter nights.

## ( **77** ) Slather on the shea butter

Get tough on dry legs with shea butter. It's a natural fat that protects skin from dehydration and other climatic influences. The linoleic acid aids cellular renewal and restores natural moisture to dry skin. Follow cleansing with a rich shea-butter–based cream before you dry off to seal in moisture, leaving your stems smooth.

## (78) A friend can help you lose weight

Research from the North American Association for the Study of Obesity says that if you have someone to check in with about your progress, you are likely to lose twice as much weight as someone who doesn't. So have a friend watch your back(side).

## (79) Look perkier

Instead of shlumping around during your weekend chores, give your face a wake-up call. Don't use the usual black eyeliner and mascara. Try white liner on your inner lower lid to brighten your eyes. Then finish with a coat of navy-blue mascara to make the whites of your eyes instantly brighter.

# (**80**) Mist me!

Nothing says long and lean better than a pair of tan legs. For a quick fix, try a misting tanning booth—a sort of color car wash. In three minutes, you will have all-over color. And not only does the fine mist create a lasting, healthy tan in under 60 seconds, it gets into all the nooks and crannies that self-tanning creams may miss. After putting a protective cream on your hands and feet, you will step into a booth, close the door, and stand in one of two positions (the operator will instruct you beforehand). After the five-second spray of color, you will turn around and stand in the other position. After the final five-second spray, you'll towel off the excess and *voilà!* The average price is $20, and the look lasts long enough to get you through the next work week.

# (81) Looking to liposuction

This is not a substitute for overall weight loss, nor is it an effective treatment for cellulite, but it can help you when it seems that nothing else will. Liposuction (lipoplasty) is particularly well-suited to women and men who are of relatively normal weight but who have isolated pockets of fat (for example, those unsightly saddlebags). Fat is removed by first inserting a small, hollow tube (a cannula) through one or more tiny incisions near the area to be suctioned. Incisions are usually less than one-quarter inch in length and are placed as inconspicuously as possible, often within skin folds or contour lines. The cannula is connected by tubing to a vacuum pressure unit. Guided by the surgeon, the suction device literally vacuums away the unwanted fat.

At what age you have it done doesn't matter as much as the condition of your skin. You will get the best results if your skin still has enough elasticity to achieve a smooth contour following fat removal. If the skin doesn't redrape well, a tightening procedure may be necessary. Areas of the body commonly treated with liposuction include hips, thighs, stomach, and buttocks, along with inner knees, calves, and ankles.

## DISCUSS WITH YOUR SURGEON BEFORE A PROCEDURE:

• Your medical history, including past and current medications and any
health problems you are having or have experienced.

• Surgical benefits, risks, and alternatives.

• Total cost, including surgeon fees, anesthesia, the facility, and others.

• Your surgeon's policy on reversionary procedures.

• Post surgical care and typical timelines for resuming work or social activities.

## FINDING A QUALIFIED PLASTIC SURGEON:

• Check with individual states for license information.

• Get info from www.abplsurg.org, the American Board of Plastic Surgery
(215-587-9322); a doctor's certification from this organization ensures
in-depth plastic surgical training.

• Visit www.surgery.org for the American Society for Aesthetic Plastic Surgery (888-272-7711); membership in this society means that a surgeon is ABPS-certified and has significant experience in cosmetic surgery for both face and body.

## RECOVERY FOR LIPOSUCTION:

Recovery can be painful, but most people are back to work within 10 days. Here is a brief breakdown of what to expect, although all cases are different.

**Swelling:** 2 weeks to 2 months

**Bruising:** 2 days to 2 weeks

**Numbness:** Several weeks

**Bandages:** Changed in 1 to 2 days, drains and sutures are removed during the first 5 to 10 days

**Work:** Return after 1 to 3 weeks

**Exercise:** Wait 2 to 4 weeks

**Final result:** Seen after 1 to 6 months

The fat will come back...just not on your butt or legs. A study by the American Academy of Dermatology found that women who had liposuction on their abs, hips, and thighs also ended up with bigger breasts (average was a cup size) two to six months post-op. They aren't sure why, but it might have something to do with an increased amount of estrogen or the fact that lipo changes a body's fat distribution.

# ( 82 ) It's time to act vein

Besides cellulite, the most common leg issue that plagues women is
visible veins, from the tiny spider to the painful varicose. But worry not.
They are treatable and sometimes even preventable.

**SPIDER VEINS:** Tiny purple veins visible through the skin

**How to treat them:** Try sclerotherapy. Most people see a 50 to 90 percent

improvement with this method, where doctors inject a saline or detergent

solution that causes the veins to collapse and disappear. The procedure

can cost around $250 per treatment and requires about three treatments

for optimal results.

**VARICOSE VEINS:** Bigger veins that bulge from underneath the skin

**How to treat them:** For those not treatable with sclerotherapy, lasers

can be used to heat and destroy the veins. There is also a procedure called radio frequency closure, where a small catheter is inserted into the defective vein using a local anesthetic. Energy is delivered through the catheter to the vein wall, causing it to shrink and seal shut. Closure costs up to $2,500 and may be covered by insurance.

Leg veins are generally hereditary, but your lifestyle can certainly add to your potential for getting them. Here are few ways to avoid them:

• Maintain a healthy weight. Extra pounds put more pressure on the veins.

• Elevate your legs after a long day on your feet, preventing blood from pooling in the legs.

• Mix up high- and low-impact activities during your exercise regimen.

• Don't keep your legs crossed for long periods of time. The best way to sit is with your ankles crossed to the side or underneath your seat. This allows good circulation through your legs while sitting.

• Wear support hose. The constriction of the tighter nylon stimulates circulation and almost makes your legs feel like they're being massaged.

## Get hair free

Whether it's for showing off in short-shorts or hidden under a pair of casual khakis, keep legs smooth with any of these defuzzing options:

## (83) Laser hair removal

In 2002, this ranked the fourth most common surgical procedure for

women, according to the American Society for Aesthetic Plastic Surgery.

The laser emits beams of light that are absorbed by the pigment in the hair.

The light is transformed into heat that destroys the hair follicle. It costs

$500 a session for a full leg, and you may need three or four sessions. This

works best on those with light skin and dark hair. If your hair is too light,

the process won't work because the laser is attracted to the pigment. For

best results, avoid waxing or shaving before the treatment.

# $\left(84\right)$ Waxing

Hot wax adheres to hairs and hardens, then is pulled off with a strip of cloth placed over the area. Home waxing products have gotten much easier to use, so don't be too shy to try it yourself. The results last three to six weeks. It costs $60 to $75 for both full legs at a salon, or $10 to $20 for at-home kits.

# $\left(85\right)$ Electrolysis

This permanent hair removal works on all skin and hair colors. The process involves inserting a tiny needle into the opening of a follicle and releasing a radiowave (thermolysis), a small electric galvanic current (traditional electrolysis), or a combination of the two. It costs $25 to $100 per hour, and you will definitely need several sessions per leg.

## ( 86 ) Depilatories

These are creams or liquids used to remove hair from the skin's surface.

Their high acid content dissolves hair in 5 to 15 minutes. Be aware that

depilatories can cause allergic reactions, are messy to apply, and some-

times have an unpleasant smell. The results last two weeks, and it costs

about $7.

## ( 87 ) Shaving

This is the easiest, quickest, and most inexpensive hair removal method,

but stubble appears quickly and ingrown hairs are a painful possibility.

Also, it only last two days. The minimal cost is the biggest benefit.

## 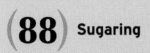 **Sugaring**

With this Egyptian method, a paste made primarily of sugar is applied to the surface of the skin and then removed with a pressed-on cloth strip. Results usually last four to six weeks. It costs around $30 to have half a leg done and $60 for a full leg.

## Fitness Fun

# (89) Take a hike

Check out trails in your area by calling your local parks department or wildlife association, or by visit hiking sites like www.localhikes.com and www.trails.com. Scenic hiking trips can burn up to 490 calories per hour. The uphill and downhill movement works your thighs and glutes better than a flat trek does.

Take along these hiking essentials to ensure that your legs get a workout that's both fun and safe.

- A day pack
- A pocket knife
- Drinking water (at least 2 liters for a day hike)
- A first-aid kit
- A detailed map of the area
- A compass
- Sunscreen
- Foods such as energy bars, fruit, and nuts

## (90) Blister blaster

Bothered by blisters? To prevent these hot spots, apply an antiperspirant (a spray or stick) to your feet for a few days in a row before your next big hike. Army researchers in Aberdeen, Maryland, found that reducing sweat decreases skin friction and cuts in half your odds of developing a blister.

## (91) Working out is a chore

Who thought that chores could actually result in more than just a clean house? Mopping, dusting, and vacuuming can give you (and your home) a workout. Housecleaning burns about 75 calories in 10 minutes. So crank up the tunes and start a tango with your broom or a samba with your vacuum.

# (92) Buy a pedometer

Studies suggest that walking 10,000 steps a day is the way to go for great leg health. Purchase a pedometer to figure out how many steps you take on an average day, and then work to add to that number. Try some of these easy ways to add steps to your 10,000-plus day:

- Instead of taking the car for short trips, throw on a pair of sneakers and walk to strengthen your lower half.
- Park as far as you can from the mall.
- Combine window-shopping with a brisk walk.
- Instead of taking the elevator or escalator, use the stairs.

Mall walking and "speed shopping" are perfect bad-weather workouts. (And shopping for that perfect little something can be a reward for your hard leg work.) If you're carrying packages on the way back to the car, that's an added bonus.

# workbook

## ( 93 ) Exercise while watching TV

Don't let a John Hughes movie marathon and a rainy day get between you and great legs and glutes. Here are a few leg exercises for an afternoon in front of the tube:

- **While lying on the floor in front of the television,** place a pillow between your knees and squeeze together. Hold for five seconds. Do this inner thigh squeeze for a count of 20.

- **Do leg lifts** while lying on the floor. Lie on your side and raise your top leg, repeat 20 times, then roll over and work the other leg.

- **Use the commercials to your advantage** with the sofa squat. Sit up on the couch with your abs tight, head neutral, and chest lifted. With feet shoulder-width apart, lean forward slightly and exhale as you push through you heels to standing. Then use your leg muscles to control your descent, as you inhale slowly. Repeat throughout the commercial break.

## (94) Bath stretches

While relaxing in the tub, stretch your legs out in front of you. Slowly
lean forward toward your toes, moving deeper into the stretch as you
slowly exhale. The warm water keeps your muscles limber. Mix in some
Dead Sea salts, which are said to have the highest concentration of
active minerals that help soothe your skin, and bring life to your aching
hamstrings and calves.

## (95) Wake without an alarm clock

Not only does being overtired give you bags under your eyes, but it can
add (saddle)bags to your butt. Studies have determined that a lack of
sleep can cause weight gain. By not getting the recommended amount,
your levels of leptin (the hormone that tells you when you're full)
decrease and your levels of the stress hormone cortisol (what makes you

hungry and directs fat to be stored in your middle) increase. So turn off that alarm clock, and wake naturally. You need an average of eight hours of sleep each night, according to the U.S. National Sleep Foundation.

# (96) Cycling

Grab a helmet and a CD of your favorite tunes, and hit the road before you start your day. Bicycling is a great lower-body workout, and soaking up the scenery is a fun way to begin a weekend. Cycling at 9 mph can burn from 315 to 480 calories an hour and really works your front thigh muscles. You can even incorporate your calf and shin muscles with toe clips, as you pull up on the clip with each spin around. Your cycling session should always begin with several knee bends and gentle stretches for your quads, hips, back, and neck.

# (97) Fight the Boogie Man

Make trips down to the basement. Climbing stairs gives you an excellent butt and thigh workout. Add a big boost to your glutes and burn even more calories by carrying your laundry along as extra weight.

# (98) Turn to the tube

Who knew that watching TV could be a great workout? Check your TV listings for follow-along aerobic exercise routines on the health and fitness channels. You can usually find morning weight workouts or yoga sessions, and they're all as close to you as your remote. Or pop in a videotape or DVD of your own. Check out step aerobics, kickboxing, or dance programs if you're looking to hit your inner and outer thighs, as well as your butt and quads.

# (99) Climb to new heights

For cuter glutes, you need to take things "up" a notch, whether it's outside (stadium stairs) or at the gym (inclined treadmill). The combo of lifting your body upward (fighting gravity every step of the way) while propelling it forward is what firms and deflabs your butt. Follow this 35-minute workout for a better bottom. It burns about 200 calories.

| Time | Walk This Way |
|---|---|
| 5 minutes | Warm up at a moderate pace. |
| 5 to 8 minutes | Steady upward climb for three flights (or a 10 to 15 percent incline). Push off with your toes and keep your buttocks tucked under. At the top of the third flight, walk down slowly (lower your treadmill to flat). Repeat as many times as you can, until you can climb for a total of 25 minutes. |
| 5 minutes | Cool down at a moderate pace by walking on a flat surface. |

# (100) Get lean muscles from stretches

Elongate your leg muscles with stretching. Each of these stretches should be held for 15 to 30 seconds without bouncing.

- **Groin.** Sit with the soles of your feet pressed together and pulled in close to your body. Lean forward, keeping your back straight.

- **Calf.** Face a wall, standing three feet away. Place your palms against the wall and lean toward it. Move one foot closer to the wall, keeping both heels on the ground. Lean forward, bending your front knee and placing your forearms against the wall. Hold, then switch legs.

- **Hamstrings.** Sit on the floor with your right leg extended. Bend your left knee and bring the sole of that foot to the inside of your right knee. Bend forward from your lower back, going only as far as is comfortable, reaching toward your right foot. Hold, then switch legs.

- **Hips and Butt.** Sit on the floor with your left leg straight. Bend your right knee and cross it over your left leg, placing your right foot flat on the floor along the outside of your left knee. Place your left elbow on the outside of your right knee. Slowly twist to the right, applying force to your right knee. Hold, then switch sides.

- **Quads.** Stand on your right leg and bend your left leg backward at the knee. With your left hand, pull up on your left ankle to stretch your quad. Hold, then switch legs.

# (101) Shoot some hoops

Nothing tones your calves (and your ego, when there's nothing but net) like a series of jump shots that would make Michael Jordan proud. If you don't have a hoop in your neighborhood, try a local YMCA or gym. The jumping motion works your calves and thighs, not to mention the shoulder workout you get as you pass the ball to win the game.

## (102) Pretend you're a kid

Start off the day with a few childish games. They will work out the right muscles and reverse the fingerprints of time that seem to be all over your butt.

**Jump rope** This childhood favorite is actually a killer cardio workout that sculpts your calves and thighs. Do it up to four times a week. If you keep getting tangled in the real thing, let your imagination run wild and just do the motions. For a real cardio kick, try it for 10 minutes.

**Jumping jacks** Works your quads, calves, and butt for a lean look. Start doing them for a minute and work up to 10 minutes to really get your heart racing.

# (**103**) Put your feet up

Stay in Friday night, put your feet up on a few pillows, and flip through your favorite magazine or catch up on your letter writing. Raising your feet above your heart on the coffee table or couch will aid in your legs' circulation and help stave off varicose veins.

# (**104**) Trainer's tips

- Stand tall with your abs pulled in tight before you start any exercise.
- Recruit more muscle fibers by mentally focusing on the body part you are working.
- Move your target muscles through their full range of motion.
- If your posture or form gets sloppy, switch to a lighter weight.

# ( 105 ) Yoga workout

With all the weekend running around—it's nice to quiet and calm the mind.
And the static positions of yoga also work your legs and butt. Try these
poses to engage your lower half, along with your mind and spirit.

**Triangle Pose.** Stand tall with your feet wide apart. Turn your right foot in

and your left foot out. Stretch your arms parallel to the floor. Bend at

your waist to the left, facing forward and placing your left hand on your left

shin as your right arm reaches straight up. Turn your head to look up at

your right hand. Hold for 15 seconds and slowly return to your starting

position. Switch sides. Do three times on each side.

**Proud Warrior.** Step your feet a wide distance apart. Turn your right foot in

and your left foot out. Stretch your arms out parallel to the floor. Turn your

head to the left as you bend your left knee to a 90-degree angle. Don't bend

your leg too far; you should be able to see your left big toe. Hold for 15 seconds, then slowly return to your starting position. Switch sides.

**Forward Bend.** Stand tall, with your arms reaching over your head. Bend forward, with your arms sweeping forward to the floor in front of your feet. Stretch your hamstrings as you hold for 15 seconds.

**Downward Dog.** From Forward Bend, step both feet back so they're about three feet from your hands, creating an inverted V shape. Stretch the backs of your legs as you pull your weight down through your heels.

## YOGA DOS AND DON'TS:

**Do take a moment to clear your mind** and get in touch with your body.

**Don't hold your breath.** Inhale and exhale deeply through your nose.

**Do move slowly** to get the most benefit from yoga and fewer injuries.

**Do exhale "aum."** This breath comes from the three minds: Oh—from the Belly, Ah—from the Heart, and M—from the Hara (Mind). When strung together, it's the well-known chant synonymous with relaxation.

# workbook

## A weighted workout

Creating resistance with your own body weight or dumbbells will help firm your thighs, hamstrings, quads, and buttocks. Use slow and controlled movements while performing this series of exercises.

## (106) Single dumbbell plié squats

**Works the hamstrings, butt, inner thighs, and quads** Stand with your feet wider than shoulder-width apart and your toes pointed out at an angle. Hold a dumbbell in both hands and let it hang in front of you. Keep your torso upright while moving downward as if you were lowering yourself into a chair until your thighs are nearly parallel with the floor. Do three sets of 10 to 12 reps.

**Tips:** Don't allow your knees to extend over your toes and keep your torso tight and erect.

# $\left(107\right)$ Stiff-legged deadlifts

**Works the hamstrings, butt, and back** Stand with your feet a little less than shoulder-width apart. Grip a bar with your hands shoulder-width apart, bending from your waist and keeping a slight bend in your knees. Keeping your back straight and your knees bent, lift the bar by straightening your back to an upright position. Slowly return the weight back down toward the ground.

**Tip:** Tighten your butt and hamstrings as you pull your torso back to the starting position. Or try propping your toes up on a board to trigger the glutes.

## ( 108 ) Leg sweeps

**Works the inner thighs** Stand with your feet hip-width apart and hands on your hips. Lift your right heel so that you are balanced on your right toe. Sweep your right leg across your body as high as you feel comfortable. Hold a moment at the top of the movement before lowering to the start. Do 10 to 12 reps; then switch legs.

## ( 109 ) Stand and curl

**Works the hamstrings** Stand with your feet about a stride's length apart. Hold on to the back of a chair. Bend your left knee slightly and lift your left heel so that you are balanced on your pointed toe. Place your hands on your hips. Bend your right knee and move your heel toward your butt. Lower to the start. Do three sets of 10 to 12 reps each side.

# (110) Pizza party

Go ahead, grab a slice! An Italian study in the *International Journal of Cancer* shows that pizza eaters (those who eat one slice or more per week) reduced their risk for certain cancers by as much as 59 percent. Instead of two slices of cheese pizza, opt for two slices of veggie pizza with no cheese. This can cut up to 150 calories and 12 grams of fat. And in our low-carb world, toss the crust.

# (111) Cut it up

Cut up veggies and fruits and place them in colorful containers in the fridge. This makes them easy alternatives to those salty and sweey stay-at-home weekend cravings that can add pounds to your hips and thighs.

# ( 112 ) Juice up your day

Need a little help on a lazy Sunday afternoon? Sip 100 percent fruit juice. The fluid and carbs add just the right amount of get-up-and-go. But steer clear of juices that contain sugar as the first ingredient (those sneaky hidden calories). Good grabs are orange (pulp for fiber), red grapefruit (lycopene to fight disease), and cranberry (for urinary tract health). Dilute with flat or sparkling water to lighten the calorie load.

# ( 113 ) You better shop around

When grocery shopping, nutritionists recommend shopping the outer aisles of the supermarket, where the more nutritious and lower-fat foods are. After filling your cart with fruits, veggies, seafood, and dairy, take a quick run through the inner aisles for anything you might have missed. (And no, that doesn't mean a visit to the chip aisle.)

# ( **114** ) Don't buy it

If it's not there, you won't eat it. Leave the chips, cakes, and cookies at the grocery store. This makes your house what experts call a "no-fail environment." That's a great place to start when keeping up with a leg-and-butt-thinning diet.

# ( **115** ) A burger without a bun?

Treat your burger like a steak and use a fork. Bypassing the bun will lower your carb and fat intake, which can mean smaller buns of your own. Although it's a little high in sugar, you can't beat ketchup for an antioxidant lypocene kick, so dab on a little. Now if we could just keep away from those fries…

# (116) Movie treats are not taboo

Ahhhh…a Saturday night at the movies. Dragging a date to a chick flick and munching on a box of popcorn the size of an oil tanker. Bad diet news, right? It doesn't have to be. The popcorn isn't the culprit; the butter and salt are. Opt for air-popped popcorn, spray with butter-flavored spray (bring your own), and add a small amount of salt. Or try a little sprinkle of parmesan cheese.

# (117) Read labels for sugar

Here's a quick trick to help you make better food choices: If the number of sugar grams is more than half of the total carbs listed, this is a high-sugar food. Put it down and walk away. The fewer the grams, the better the gams!

# ( **118** ) Protein for energy

It's important to load up on protein in the morning for a productive day full of long-lasting energy. (How else will you take full advantage of two days off?) Using egg whites, make a nice healthy omelet with fresh veggies. Add a slice of whole wheat bread for just the right amount of carbs.

## High-Energy Omelet

- 3 egg whites
- Splash of skim milk
- Nonfat cooking spray
- Veggies (onions, mushrooms, and peppers are good choices)
- Fat-free cheese

Mix the egg whites and milk together. Coat an omelet pan with cooking spray and sauté the veggies over medium heat until tender. Pour in the egg mixture. When the egg is almost cooked to your liking, sprinkle the cheese on one half. Fold over and cook until the cheese melts. Slide onto a plate and enjoy your guiltless breakfast!

# (119) Dem bones, dem bones

You heard it as a kid: "Honey, drink your milk." Well, momma wasn't kidding. If you don't have enough calcium in your diet, plan on asking, Got Osteoporosis? Osteoporosis is a disease of the skeletal system characterized by low bone mass and deterioration of bone tissue. According to the National Institute of Health, women ages 25 to 50 need 1,000 mg per day. That's four to five cups of milk, cheese, or yogurt each day. Adequate calcium can also contribute to weight loss.

# (120) Pumping the iron

Getting ready for a weekend of hard play? Add more iron to your diet. Choose iron-rich foods like shellfish, lean beef, liver, sardines, cooked dried beans, spinach, and fortified cereals. The recommended daily allowance of this important mineral is 10 to 15 mg.

# (121) Giddyap to good leg health

The herb horse chestnut has been soothing the troubled legs of beauties since the 18th century. Today's women use the seeds to promote circulation through the veins while toning them. The Archives of Dermatology reported that studies of the seed's extract brought about a major reduction in leg swelling, as well as eased the feeling of "tired, heavy legs." You can find horse chestnut supplements at health and herbal stores.

# (122) Berry berry good for you

Toss a handful of blueberries on your morning cereal or oatmeal. Packed with resveratrol, a micronutrient that reduces artery damage (meaning it's good for circulation and keeping those footsies warm), they are also a great picnic partner for a weekend getaway. You should always aim for at least five servings of fruits and veggies a day. Other good sources of resveratrol: red grapes, plums, and cranberries.

# (123) According to the experts...

Go ahead and dress in trendy cords. Just choose fine-wale looks to get the texture without the added bulk. As an added bonus, corduroy gives you lots of vertical lines, so you look taller and your legs look longer.

# (124) Butt-boosting jeans

Believe it or not, designers are giving our butts a lift with butt-boosting jeans. They're not actually padded, but you can see the lift when you slip on a pair.

# ( 125 ) Tall girls, beware

If you're tall and you don't want to look like a giant, stay away from capris and shorter pants. Straight leg pants with no pleats and boot cuts work best, especially if they're paired with funky flats.

# ( 126 ) Oversize handbag

Sounds too good to be true, but proportion can play tricks on the eye, making your butt actually appear smaller. When you reach for a purse, pick a shape that flatters (square shapes complement a rounder figure) and a strap length that doesn't land in a problem area (don't let the bottom of the purse rest on full hips).

# workbook

## Weekend jeans

It's easy to put on a pair of jeans for lounging around, but nothing's harder than finding a pair that flatters you. Pair the perfect pair with high-heeled boots or flat sneakers, depending on where your days off take you. And remember, don't paint on your jeans. Too-tight jeans will make you look even bigger than you are and draw attention to your thighs and butt. Find yourself in the list below and get ready to shop for newer, more flattering denim.

## ( 127 ) Too-big rear

Always buy a lower-riding pair of jeans. High-waist styles just create a wall

of fabric behind you. Styles with a relaxed fit are just perfect. Avoid small

pockets, which can make your butt look bigger. The right look puts pockets

right in the middle of your backside.

# ( 128 ) Too-prominent hips

Choose generously cut styles, as they won't call attention to your bigger hips. Try a slightly flared bottom (and I do mean slightly) to even out the proportions.

# ( 129 ) Too-short legs

To lengthen legs, invest in a pair of jeans with a narrow straight-leg or boot-cut style, both of which elongate the leg. These look perfect with high-heeled boots. To add even more inches, make sure the hem of your jeans reaches mid-heel.

# ( 130 ) Boyish figure

Buy button-front hip-huggers to accentuate your femininity. Play up curves with contrast topstitching and higher-set pockets. Stay away from anything too tight that might make your legs look like skinny sticks. A bit of stretch is an advantage, but stay away from anything too stretchy.

# ( 131 ) Pear-shaped

One-third of all women are pear-shaped. You may be tempted to wear baggy jeans in an attempt to hide those thighs, but you should really try wearing fitted jeans to streamline that figure. People with fuller lower halves should also avoid peg-legged jeans (leave them in the '80s).

# $\left(132\right)$ Full-figured

Choose jeans that follow the shape of your body but don't hug every curve. A pair of relaxed, medium-waist jeans with straight legs is your safest bet.

# ( **133** ) Did you know?

The butts covered in the blue stuff were a little less cute and feminine in the 18th century. Trade laborers and plantation workers once donned denim for its hardiness. It wasn't until the late 19th century that the first pair of riveted jeans were patented and marketed by Levi Strauss.

# ( **134** ) Never wear faded denim

Acid-washed denim has—thankfully—not reared its ugly head (or butt) since the '80s, but lighter colored jeans in general aren't the most flattering. Deep, dark denim is the most slimming and will make you look like you dropped five pounds instantly.

# (135) Low-rise panty tip

It makes sense—low-cut underwear for under low-rise jeans. Practice bending over in front of a mirror to make sure that your unmentionables aren't mentioned over the top of your jeans.

# (136) It's all in the fit

Choose clothes that fit you. Don't go larger, because it will exaggerate your size rather than hiding it. Elyse Jacob, owner of Kartel Kollections, says clothing should skim the flesh for the perfect fit. You should feel it touch your hips and butt, but it shouldn't hug. If it's too tight it will create dimples, making you look like you are squeezed in and heavier than you are.

## (137) Avoid a saggy seat

Jeans that gently hug your hips are always more flattering. Pick a stretch denim to eliminate a saggy seat and provide extra comfort.

## (138) Wrap it up

Wrap a short, thin, shawl around your hips at an angle over your jeans. This will create a vertical sight line away from your butt, smoothing out your figure and giving length to your legs.

## (139) Contrasting proportions

Don't make the mistake of going for all long or all short pieces. Contrast proportions, mixing a longer jacket with a shorter skirt or a shorter jacket with pants. This will create length and thin out your body.

# workbook

## ( 140 ) Casual pants

When choosing casual slacks that are a cut above jeans for a business-casual afternoon, try these tips:

· **If you need a lift in the butt,** try thick fabrics for control, plus look for fool-the-eye high pockets.

· **If you have saddlebags**, skip the stretch fabrics. Wear brocade or anything that's not clingy.

· **If you're big,** go for low-rise pants in a dark color.

· **If you have short legs,** don't cuff your pants. The cuff can make your legs seem cut off and stumpy.

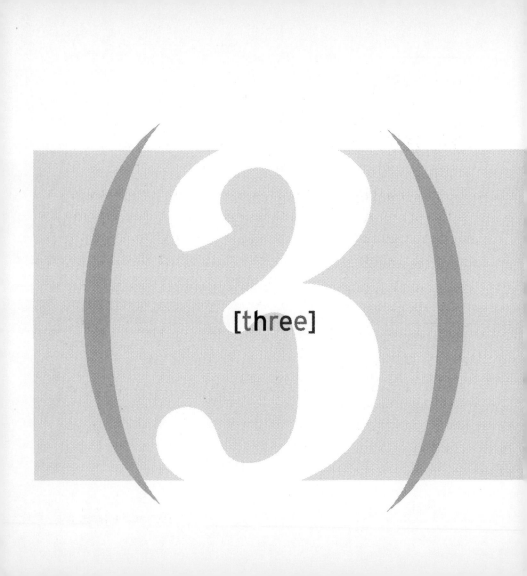

(3)

[three]

# Beach Blanket Beauty

**There's no way to hide anything on the beach.**
Certainly not behind the itsy-bitsy teeny-weenie
fashions that have wiggled their ways onto the butts of
today's sun worshipers. It seems that cellulite, fat on
your fanny, and any tiny blemishes are all magnified
under the summer sun. It's a spotlight for flaws that
normally hide under pants or skirts. But relax. After
you follow these tips there will be no more shrieking
from the dressing room when you try on the latest
two-piece. This chapter will help you minimize the
flab, give your skin a healthy sun-kissed look (yes, it's
possible!), and ensure that nothing is sagging behind

you while you stroll the sand dunes. And with a butt and legs like you'll boast, the umbrella in your piña colada won't be the only thing causing a stir. ~

# (141) Trade in dull skin for glowing skin

Over your lifetime, you will shed some 90 pounds of dead skin—yuck. Exfoliate dull legs and bums with this homemade summery citrus scrub. Mix a paste out of $1/2$ to $2/3$ cup granulated sugar and the juice of one lemon. While showering, invigorate your skin with the paste. Use the inside of the lemon rind to rub heels and elbows. And blondes, save a little lemon juice to put on your hair at the beach for a sun-kissed shine.

## ( **142** ) Protect the backs of your legs

Don't forget to apply sunscreen to the backs of your legs and behind your knees. Most people neglect these areas of their legs, so this is one of the most common places for skin cancer due to sunburn. Besides, you want people staring at your butt because it's hot, not because it's on fire.

## ( **143** ) Spray your way to smooth skin

Body mists and sprays are excellent ways to hydrate and refresh your parched legs after bathing or sun exposure. Choose mists that nourish the skin with plant and herb essences, such as soothing aloe vera.

## ( **144** ) Slim your legs with seaweed

Seaweed wraps release water retention and leave legs looking their sleekest! Soak your legs in a bath of warm water and Epsom salts for 5 minutes. Pat dry. Apply a seaweed mask (such as BlissLabs' High Thighs Seaweed Task Mask), then wrap legs with plastic wrap and a warm towel. Relax for 15 minutes. Remove the towel and plastic wrap and rinse your legs clean.

## ( **145** ) Add a little salt

Shake a little sea salt into your bath. It reverses water retention, detoxifies cells, and banishes bloating. Rub a little onto your legs as a mild abrasive scrub. Its water solubility allows it to dissolve while you're using it, so there's no sticky leftover mess.

# (146) Enjoy a sand witch

Dab on a little witch hazel to calm leg irritations from sunburn, insect bites, poison ivy, rashes, and stings. Thousands of Native American women can't be wrong. And in Europe, an extract derived from witch hazel is taken internally to soothe leg veins. You can find witch hazel at most stores that carry health and beauty products.

# (147) Make an appointment with a dermatologist

Make sure all your moles are regular in shape and color and haven't grown over the years. And don't forget to look between your toes! According to studies, people spot 75 percent of melanomas themselves, but that doesn't get you out of an annual dermatologist visit. Look for new growths that are pink, red, black, or dark brown; pay attention to growths that are flat or raised.

## ( **148** ) Soothing aloe vera

Smooth skin with aloe before and after sun exposure. Aloe will hydrate sun-worshipping skin and its anti-inflammation agents will help heal any sun damage. Grow a plant of your own, cut off a bit of the stalk, split it in half, and rub the clear goo on your legs.

## ( **149** ) Sunless tanning

Although avoided by today's smart bathing beauties, the first intentional tan was sported by Coco Chanel in the 1930s. If you crave the cocoa color but shun the sun, give sunless tanning creams and sprays a try. With light creams and user-friendly sprays, these tanners are a girl's best friend. Follow these tips for a streak-free, natural-looking tan:

1. For great results, exfoliate with a scrub before you apply.
2. Use an oil-free moisturizer on your skin before you apply the tanner. (Oil will cause streaks and uneven application.)

3. Use long, even strokes to apply. Work from top to bottom. Try to mimic the long, smooth motions of the professional massage therapist.

4. You want it to look natural, so be wary of putting a lot on your knees, ankles, wrists, and elbows, where creases can occur.

5. Wash your hands immediately after applying the tan.

6. Let the tanner dry for a few minutes, then buff yourself all over with an old sock turned inside out. Use small circular motions to ensure evenness.

7. Wait at least 10 to 15 minutes before you put on clothes.

# (150) Healing sands

It's no wonder that Brazilian women are ready to bare it all (à la the Brazilian wax). They rub sand on their bodies to break up cellulite. When lying on the beach, grab a handful and start to rub it on any spots that are troublesome, like the backs of your thighs and butt cheeks. (Be inconspicuous, though; this could look a little weird to beachgoers.)

# ( 151 ) Apply sunscreen before you leave

Prep your skin at least 30 minutes before you start sunbathing to allow the sunscreen to be fully absorbed. Don't go lower than SPF 15. According to a study from the FDA, you will get only 23 percent of your total UV exposure by the time you're 18, not the 80 percent originally thought, so it's never too late for SPF.

# ( 152 ) Cellulite madness

It's the bane of every butt's existence—would you believe that 90 percent of all women have cellulite? As we gain weight, our fat cells swell while our connective tissues (what connects fat to skin) stay the same, thereby causing that lovely dimpling effect. You can minimize that bumpy behind with the following tips:

- Eat well and avoid salty foods.
- Drink lots of water.
- Exercise.

# ( 153 ) Take care of your skin

Anti-cellulite creams, while not able to get rid of cellulite long-term, do hydrate or swell the skin with ingredients like caffeine, ginseng, and soy, smoothing it temporarily. To apply, first dry brush your legs, then exfoliate for two to three minutes in a circular motion. This will help your skin absorb the active ingredients faster. Apply the cellulite cream from below your knees to the top of your bottom. Good lines to try are BlissLabs' thigh serums and scrubs, and Neutrogena's Anti-Cellulite Treatment with Retinol.

# ( 154 ) See a specialist

For severe cellulite, or when you've tried everything else, there are professional procedures that have shown some success. During these treatments (quite pricey at around $525 to $1,050), a trained specialist runs the head of the endermologie machine (rollers connected to a powerful vacuum) over the area, providing an intense massage that breaks up the cellulite.

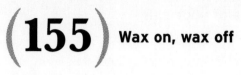

# ( **155** ) Wax on, wax off

Waxing to get rid of unwanted hair on your lower half goes hand-in-hand with the beach and the season's small summer suits.

**Here's how it's done:** A tongue depressor or spatula is used to spread a thin layer of wax over skin in the direction of hair growth. A cloth strip is pressed onto the wax and then ripped off with a quick movement. When all is said and done you'll have smooth, hairless skin for three to six weeks. It costs $60 to $75 to have both legs done at a salon or spa, or $25 to $40 for just the bikini area. At-home waxing kits (available for $10 to $20) are a great, easy option.

# ( **156** ) That makes scents

Soothe the sting during leg or bikini waxing with a vanilla candle. A University of Quebec study in the *Journal of Physiology and Behavior* found that women's pain receptors respond favorably to certain smells, decreasing sensations of pain.

# ( **157** ) Wax to the max

Follow these dos and don'ts for both salon experiences and trips to your own bathroom "spa."

- Don't wax during your period. Your body has a lower threshold for pain during this time.
- Do grow hair to at least $\frac{1}{8}$ inch long before waxing.
- Do rub in the same direction as the hair growth when applying the strip over the wax.
- Do pull the skin taut before pulling the cloth off.
- At a salon, do make sure the strips of cloth aren't being reused.

# ( **158** ) Spray water on your legs

When planning a lazy sun day, bring a small plant mister full of water. Spray your legs periodically for a glistening look. The water with hydrate your skin and the reflected light makes your legs look firmer.

# (159) Bounce up and down

You're hitting the beach, so why not start off having a ball? Grab your sturdy beach ball (or exercise balance ball) and bounce up and down on it for five to ten minutes. This will tone your legs and glutes, and let's face it, it's fun.

# (160) While you lounge

While lying ocean-side, squeeze that butt! Think of lifting your glutes up and back, as if you were holding a dollar between them. A quick work-out tip worth a million.

# (161) An indoor water workout

Everybody into the pool! Water aerobics is a great way to increase your strength and flexibility. A typical water workout lasts 50 minutes and burns 450 to 700 calories. The lower body gets the most benefit, from kicks, leg extensions, squats, knee lifts, walking, marching, and jogging. Check you local gyms or YMCAs for class times, then show off your results along the shores of the world's biggest outdoor pool.

# (162) Elliptical trainer

Walk, step, ski, and cycle all at once? Enter the elliptical trainer. With smoother movements than a stair stepper, it's nicer to your knees, but it works your butt, hamstrings, and quads mercilessly. Plan on burning up to a whopping 750 calories an hour. Choose an elliptical trainer with dual action that links arm motion to foot movement. You'll burn more calories and get a great upper body workout.

# ( **163** ) Step to it

Stepping up builds shapely legs and glutes. A step bench (one that adjusts) can provide high-intensity aerobic exercise that you will feel for days afterwards. Look for one that comes with an instructive videotape; prices range from around $25 to $85.

Put aside 30 minutes, give the following routine a try on a high step (10 to 12 inches), and say goodbye to around 320 calories. Make sure not to bend your knees so that they go beyond your toes. Begin and end with five minutes of basic stepping up and down (see below) at an easy intensity level. Cycle through the following step moves.

**1. Basic step:** Step up with your right foot, then with your left. Step down with your right foot, then with your left. After 8 reps, tap your left toe on floor and step up with your left foot, repeating reps on opposite side.

**2. Knee lift:** Step up with your right foot, then bring your left leg in front of you, bending your left knee up to 90 degrees. Step down with your left foot, then tap your right toe on the floor and step up with your right foot again to repeat. After 8 reps, switch legs and step up with your left foot, lifting your right knee.

**3. Step-up and kick:** Follow the directions for Knee Lift, but kick your foot out in front of you at a 45-degree angle instead of lifting your knee to 90 degrees. Perform 8 times on each side.

**4. Hamstring curl:** Follow the directions for Knee Lift, but bend your left knee to curl your heel towards your buttocks. After 8 reps on each side, return to the knee lift move and cycle through for the remaining 20 minutes.

# ( **164** ) Different day, different workout

Celebrity trainer Michael George trains his clients using a technique he calls Integrated Motivational Fitness. To keep it interesting, he suggests doing a different cardio activity every day of the week. That way, you won't burn out your muscles—or your attention span.

**Monday.** Take a step or low-impact aerobic class for balance and agility.

**Tuesday.** Work the machines: 15 minutes on the treadmill, 15 minutes on the elliptical trainer, and 15 minutes on the bicycle for a well-rounded leg and butt workout.

**Wednesday.** Choose a new activity; maybe try the belly dancing or hip-hop dance class at your gym.

**Thursday.** Participate in a sports league or pick-up game.

**Friday.** Take a swim for a low-impact, high-calorie-burning workout. Choose strokes with kicks for good leg motion.

**Saturday.** Unwind from the week with a yoga class to increase flexibility and decrease stress.

**Sunday.** Take it outside for biking, hiking, or walking.

# ( **165** ) Breaking up is good to do

Research shows that you'll burn the same amount of calories whether you do your workout all at once or in bits and pieces. Do a brisk 10-minute walk up and down your apartment stairs before the beach, walk the dunes for 10 minutes that afternoon, then bop to your favorite tunes for 10 minutes while you're unpacking your beach bag at home.

# ( **166** ) Stair climber workout

One of the best machines for your calves, thighs, and glutes, climbers can help you burn 500 calories per hour. Use correct posture, standing up straight and keeping your upper body in the same vertical plane as your hips and legs. Don't lean over the climber, and don't support your body with your arms on the handlebars. Start at a lower step rate and work up to mountains from molehills.

## ( **167** ) Check your walk

To get the most out of your walking workout, make sure that you roll each hip forward to buffer the impact. Your heel should touch the ground and you should push off with your big toe. For a good walking workout, rate your exertion using a scale from 1 to 10, with 1 meaning relaxed and 10 meaning thoroughly exhausted. Start at level 2 or 3, working up to level 6 to 8, and then cooling down to level 2.

## ( **168** ) Walk, don't run

Running on the beach can be tough on your Achilles tendon because your foot keeps sinking down once it hits the ground and your leg is pulling back up. Try walking instead.

# ( **169** ) Don't workout too close to bedtime

Exercise one or two hours before you turn in. Exercising too close to bedtime can lead to a bad night's sleep and possibly midnight leg cramps. But aerobic exercise at the right time helps you fall asleep an average of 12 minutes faster and helps you sleep 42 minutes longer than nonexercisers, according to a Stanford University study.

# ( **170** ) Doorknob squats

Set a timer to 100 seconds. Stand facing the narrow edge of an open door with your legs hip-distance apart and a footstool directly behind you. Grip one doorknob in each hand. To a slow count of 10, lower your body until your bottom touches the stool—but don't sit down. Pause, then raise yourself to a standing position to another slow count of 10. Repeat until the time is up.

# (171) In with the good air...

Fuel your muscles by breathing. If you hold your breath, your muscles suffer and become fatigued sooner. Inhale, expand your lungs, and expel the breath fully.

Try these breathing techniques while you have the fresh ocean air at your disposal:

1. **Kihap** (a martial arts technique that dampens stress): Inhale through your nose and exhale through your mouth, gradually exhaling louder as you breathe from your diaphragm.

2. **Belly** (combats sluggishness): Lie on your back with your feet flat and knees bent. Place your hands on top of each other over your navel. Feel your belly rise and fall. Press gently while exhaling.

3. **Humming** (quiets the mind and muscles with vibrations): Inhale through your nose, keeping your mouth closed, then hum to exhale. Low pitches work best.

# workbook

## ( 172 ) Get a Brazilian (body, not wax)

**Capoeira (pronounced "cap-WEAR-ah")** is an Afro-Brazilian movement creating quite a stir in the fitness world. Perfect for achieving firmer glutes and toned legs, it blends martial arts, acrobatics, and dance—all to the beat of energized music. The routine is usually done sans shoes and in loose clothing, so turn on some lively music and feel the rhythm. Try this twice a week and say goodbye to an extra 400 calories. Do each move 8 to 16 times with no rest between reps for a great cardio session.

**Ginga (sway):** Stand with feet wider than shoulder-width. Squat slightly, with elbows bent and hands in front of your chest. Step back with your left foot and into a lunge and twist your torso slightly to the right (hips facing forward), swinging your left elbow forward and right elbow back. Return to start. Repeat on the other side.

**Esquiva (escape) to front**: Begin in the Ginga position. In one motion, lunge to the left, foot angled out (don't let your knee go past your toes) and twist your lower torso so your chest hovers above your left knee. Keeping your back straight, lift your bent arms out to each side at about shoulder height. Return to start. Repeat on the other side.

**Esquiva to side:** From Ginga, step forward with your left foot, turning your body to the right and looking to the left. Squat a little deeper. Keep your back straight as you lean your torso forward and lift your bent arms out to each side. Return to start. Repeat on the other side.

**Negativa (negative):** From Ginga, squat deeply, put your left hand on the floor, and extend your left leg forward. Bend your torso over your left thigh, right elbow up in front. Place your right hand on the floor in front of your right knee and slide your left foot back, ending with feet wide. Press your butt up to straighten your legs as much as possible, keeping your torso angled down. Return to start. Repeat on the other side.

**Bencao (blessing):** From Ginga, twist your torso slightly to the left (hips stay forward) and balance by leaning back as you lift your left knee as high as possible, bringing your left elbow back and your right elbow forward. Holding your knee up, kick your left foot out, straightening your leg as much as you can. Return to start. Repeat on the other side.

**Pisao (big step):** From Ginga, bend your torso forward, keeping your head up. (Steady yourself on a chair if necessary.) Bend your left knee and lift it to the side as high as you can, keeping your foot behind your body. Keeping your hips forward and head up, kick your left leg back, foot flexed. Return to start. Repeat on the other side.

**Negativa de Queda (negative fall):** From Ginga, squat deeply, place your right hand on the floor, and swing your right leg forward so your right thigh and calf hover just off the floor, foot flexed. Place your left hand on the floor and bend your elbows while lowering your right ear and chest close to the floor. Your torso and right leg should form a right angle. Return to start. Repeat on the other side.

**Carivete (penknife):** Lie on the floor with your knees slightly bent. Contract your abs to lift your head and torso entirely off the floor. Bring both hands up so your arms are parallel to the floor and lift your left knee in toward your chin. Lower and repeat with your right leg. Continue smoothly to exhaustion.

**THE DOS OF CAPOEIRA**

• **Do go with the flow.** Practice each move slowly, then pick up the pace as you become more comfortable.

• **Do control the motions.**

• **Do loosen up.** Warm up for 5 to 10 minutes with easy dancing or jogging in place.

• **Do have fun!**

# (173) Sprint your way to great legs

A great way to add power to your legs is to incorporate sprinting into your workout. It builds great hamstrings, glutes, and calves. Walk for 5 minutes to get warmed up, then feel the need for speed. Sprint for a minute or so, then go back to walking. Alternate for a 30-minute workout. When that becomes too easy, go for longer or add an incline.

# (174) Beach ball exercises

Have a ball toning your lower half with an exercise ball. By forcing you to balance on an unstable surface, this workout activates small muscles that don't usually get used. The ball must be strong enough to hold your weight and should be big enough to cover the length of your back. Follow these exercises for beach-going gams and glutes.

- **Quad circles:** Sit on the ball with arms outstretched for balance. Lift and straighten one leg in front of you. With your foot, make little circles in the air. Perform three sets of 12 to 15 reps on each leg.
- **Ball squeeze:** Sit on the ground and place the ball between your ankles. Lie back and grip the upper portion of the ball with your heels. Make sure your toes point straight upwards. Contract your inner thighs by pressing the ball with your heels and then lift your hips up off the floor. Hold for three seconds and release, with control.
- **Bridge hip extension:** Sit on the ball with your arms outstretched in front for balance. Lean back and walk out far enough so that your head and shoulders are supported by the ball. Keep your abdominals tight to support your back. Hold and feel the burn in your quads and glutes as you squeeze the muscles tight.
- **Abduction:** Kneel with your right hip supported by the ball, your right knee on the floor, and your left leg extended directly to the side in line with your torso. Place your right hand and arm on the ball for support. Lift your left leg up to hip height, pause, then lower. Do one to three sets of 8 to 12 reps switching sides between sets.

## ( 175 ) Jump in (the water's fine!)

Never mind running along the beach. Try running in the ocean. The resistance that the water creates will give you a challenging workout, exercising your quads, calves, and hip flexors.

## ( 176 ) Stretch for length

To lengthen your muscles, stretch every day. Do at least one stretch for every major muscle group in your body, including your butt, thighs (front and back), calves, and quads. Hold each stretch for 30 to 60 seconds. Breathe deeply and relax as you stretch. Never push beyond a point of mild discomfort, and don't stretch muscles that haven't been warmed up.

# workbook

## The power of Pilates

Pilates builds and tones the muscles of your legs and butt, along with sculpting fantastic abs by working through your strong center core. Warm up for about three minutes with a little walking or marching in place. After your workout, do three more minutes of cool down (light stretching and walking) with a bit of meditation.

## ( 177 ) Alternating leg stretch

Lay on a mat on your back. Lifting your head and shoulders off of the

mat, hold your right leg gently straight up in the air and stretch your left

leg away from you, holding it about two inches off the ground. Lift it

higher if you feel your back arching. Slowly swap the positions of your

legs, making a scissors motion as you do. Keep continuous movement

and breathe in for two changes, then out for two. Do 15 with each leg.

# (178) Side leg lifts

Lie on the floor on your left side with your legs at a 45-degree angle in front of you, head resting on your outstretched arm or on your hand. Place your palm on the floor in front of your abs for support. Align your right hip directly over your left hip and pull your abs in so your back isn't arched. Raise your right leg until your foot is directily above your shoulders. Then slowly lower your leg back down as if pushing through thick air. Repeat 15 times, then switch legs. Do three sets.

# (179) Kickback

Get down on your knees and forearms. Bend your left leg at a 90-degree angle behind you, then flex your left foot and lift it toward the ceiling.

Being careful not to move your pelvis, pulse your foot three to four inches toward the ceiling. Perform 15 reps and switch legs.

## $\left(180\right)$ One leg circles

Lie flat on the mat with your arms at your sides. Pull in your abs. Pointing your toes, stretch your left leg toward the ceiling as far as possible without straining. Rotate your left leg clockwise in a small circle, using the hip joint as the center of the clock face. Your hips should not move. Circle 10 times, then rotate counterclockwise. Switch legs.

## ( **181** ) Did you know?

Although the trends of yoga and Pilates are relatively new, they are certainly not as green as you would believe. Yoga's been around for about 5,000 years, and Pilates was developed by Joseph Pilates, with his first studio opening in New York City in the 1920s.

## ( **182** ) Anytime, anywhere

Whenever you have a chance, stretch your legs. Tying your shoe? Fold all the way over for a great hamstring stretch. When you're bending over to wrap your wet hair in a towel, when you're picking up the morning paper…there are always opportunities throughout the day when you can work toward leaner, more limber legs.

# ( **183** ) The great outdoors

Why stop at the beach? There are tons of butt-blasting outdoor activities for you to enjoy in the beautiful weather. So get the ball rolling with these suggestions:

**Go blading.** Inline skating works the butt, inner thighs, and outer thighs (so no more saddlebags).

**Take a hike.** Running or walking up hills sculpts your butt and your thighs.

**Go for a swim.** A wonderful overall leg toner, choose strokes such as the breaststroke and butterfly, which emphasize kicking.

**Play in the water.** Running in waist-deep water and aqua aerobics do a great job of chiseling your leg muscles.

## Before you hit the beach...

Put your beach blanket (and legs) to work before they find their way to the sandy dunes for a lovely lazy lounge.

# ( 184 ) Kneeling leg curl

Kneel on your elbows and knees on a thick towel, positioning your knees directly under your hips and your elbows directly under your shoulders. Clasp your hands together or turn your palms toward the floor. Flex your right foot so that it is perpendicular to the floor. Keeping your knee bent, lift your right leg and raise your knee up to hip level. Tilt your chin lightly toward your chest and pull your abs in so your back doesn't sag. Straighten your leg and then bend your knee. Complete 10 to 12 reps with one leg before switching legs.

# ( 185 ) Quad press

Roll up a small beach towel. Sit on the floor and lean against a wall with your legs straight out in front of you. Place the towel underneath your right knee. Squeeze your quads tightly and press down on the towel. Hold for five slow counts, then relax. Complete 10 to 12 reps, then switch legs.

# ( 186 ) Inner thigh lift

Lie on your right side with your head resting on your outstretched arm. Bend your left leg and rest your knee on top of a rolled-up towel, so that your knee is level with your hip and your top hip is directly over your bottom hip. Place your left hand on the floor in front of your chest for support. Pull in your abs. Lift your right (bottom) leg a few inches off the floor. Hold, then slowly lower your leg back down. Complete 10 to 12 reps before switching sides.

## (**187**) Antioxidant smoothies

Sprinkle a little wheat germ in your pre-beach smoothie for smoother legs. Chock full of selenium, known to minimize the damaging effects of ultraviolet light, this antioxidant mineral can reduce your risk of sunburn. Other nonsmoothie foods that contain selenium are garlic, tuna, whole grains, and sesame seeds.

## (**188**) Bar none

Research shows that people who replace several meals a week with portion-controlled food (such as shakes or meal replacement bars) lose more weight in three months than those who just cut calories. That makes bars the perfect beach bag snack for smaller derrieres.

## ( **189** ) Put protein in every meal

Eating protein at every meal can speed up your metabolism by as much as 25 percent, helping you burn away extra calories.

## ( **190** ) Eat fiber...but not too much

It leads to good GI tract health, weight loss, and a full tummy, so too much fiber can't be wrong, right? Not so. Eating more than you need to can cause bloat. According to the American Dietetic Association, you should limit fiber intake to no more than 10 grams at one sitting, and always drink plenty of water to help wash it down. Find it in dried fruits, shredded wheat, figs, prunes, and veggies.

# (191) Go fish

Look to the ocean for more than just a place to sun worship. The ocean is teeming with fish, and fish is reeling with B vitamins and lean protein—and some even contain omega-3 fatty acids. Aim to eat 12 ounces of fish a week. If you're buying a whole fresh fish, look for clear eyes, bright skin, and flesh that springs back when pressed. Splash it with lime juice and a little rosemary, then toss it on the grill.

# (192) Food diary

Can't understand why you are gaining weight when you are watching "exactly" what you eat? According to the *New England Journal of Medicine*, you might be kidding yourself by at least 16 percent. Start a food diary and list every single thing you eat during the day. After one week, look it over to see if you're eating as little as you think you are.

# (193) Use your food diary

You may want to cut several inches off your thighs, but don't cut too many calories off your diet—at least not all at once. Your body is programmed to defend its weight, so if you suddenly eliminate 1,000 calories, your metabolism will slow down. Instead, use your food diary to calculate your intake, then cut 500 calories from that. Never consume fewer than 1,200 calories per day.

# (194) Allow yourself a treat every so often

If you have a vice, whether it's candy, salty foods, or in my case, cheese, don't deny yourself. That will just lead to a binge later. Have a small handful of M&Ms or a cookie as a treat to yourself once or twice a week.

# ( **195** ) Have some peanut butter

Have a tablespoon of peanut butter for a snack. It's full of Vitamin E, the guardian of skin tissues. Vitamin E can also be found in wheat germ oil, vegetable and seed oils, and seeds and nuts. Try for the RDA of 400 mg.

# ( **196** ) What's up, doc?

Throw a few carrots in your beach bag for munching. German researchers have found that as little as 30 milligrams a day of the beta carotene found in carrots can help reduce the redness and inflammation of sunburn. Beta carotene accumulates in the skin and provides 24-hour protection against sun damage (but this doesn't mean you should skip the SPF). You can also find it in a few refreshing slices of watermelon—another great beach treat. Other sources are dark-colored produce such as sweet potatoes, tomatoes, broccoli, and spinach.

# ( **197** ) A bunch of mini-meals

Experts say that five or six mini-meals keep blood sugar levels balanced, boosting metabolism, and sustaining energy. A mini-meal contains between 300 and 400 calories. Some good picks for your beach cooler:

- ¾ cup high-fiber cereal with skim milk, 1 orange
- ¼ cup baby carrots dipped in hummus, 1 hard-boiled egg
- Half a basil, tomato, and mozzarella sandwich on whole wheat
- 1 chicken drumstick, a small bunch of grapes
- An 8-ounce parfait of yogurt, granola, chocolate sauce, and fruit

# ( **198** ) Spice it up

Studies have shown that eating fiery red pepper-spiced meals may increase your metabolism by up to 30 percent. Sprinkle the flakes on pizza, eggs, salads, or whatever appeals to you. What a great way to achieve hot legs!

## ( **199** ) It's easy eating greens

Have a fresh salad before your beach trip for a light, healthy meal.
Baby spinach and romaine lettuce are nutritious, they're good sources
of roughage, and they are extremely low in calories. A 10-ounce bag
of spinach has approximately 62 calories, and the same bag of romaine
has about 40 calories. Add some grilled chicken or fish with low-fat
dressing, and it's the perfect summer meal.

## ( **200** ) Don't overdo the fruit

Easy-to-pack fruit is a tempting treat for the beach, but don't overdo it.
It has calories and sugar galore! Think two a day maximum, and only
the low-sugar, high-fiber variety. Apples, pears, plums, and berries are
all good choices, and yes, no bananas!

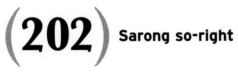

## Fashion Facts

## (201) Make sure your suit fits

Plan on going up a size when it comes to your bathing suit, but don't go too big. Saggy drawers and drooping straps add pounds to your body and make your butt look frumpy.

## (202) Sarong so-right

Try a stylish sarong worn low on the hips. It will cover the butt and thigh area and give you an island flair. The slit in the front will make your legs look longer by adding a vertical sight line.

# (203) The hats have it

Throw on a wide, floppy hat to draw attention away from your shy lower half. Your skin will also thank you for the shade.

# (204) Ankle bracelets

Thin ankle bracelets add femininity and a dainty look. They're the perfect way to bring a little sparkle to your bare beach legs. But leave the thicker anklets to the chain gangs, as they can make your ankle look too cut off and your leg bigger.

## Bathing suits

Walk proud and confident in a suit that makes you feel comfortable, sexy, and slim. Comfort leads to a better mindset. To make legs look longer and slimmer, opt for scoop, high-cut legs. Boy-cut suits are unflattering to most women, so stay away if you have larger thighs or saddlebags. Strong material like Lycra is perfect for holding in the butt. And skirted suits are also a stylish option—they're not just for grannies anymore. Follow these tips to choose the best bathing suit for your body shape.

## (205) Hourglass

**(balanced shoulders and hips, with a defined waist)**

A two-piece suit will highlight your waist and all-over prints will keep the

eyes moving.

## ( 206 ) Triangle

**(narrower shoulders and wider hips)**

An empire waist makes a small bust look fuller; since the eye is attracted to light shades, wear a paler top, possibly with horizontal stripes, and a darker, solid bottom.

## ( 207 ) Inverted triange

**(wider bust, narrower hips)**

Choose high-neck suits, underwire tops, and other suits with plenty of coverage and support; a wide, square neck narrows wide shoulders; balance things with a fuller-cut bottom, or maybe even a pair of boy shorts.

## ( 208 ) Rectangle

**(straight line from shoulder to hip; no waist)**

Look for special detailing that defines a waist, such as piping or a side

cutout; create a waist with a wide horizontal stripe around the middle.

## ( 209 ) Circle

**(balanced shoulders and hips, with a wider waist)**

Look for suits with slimming fabric in the torso to smooth the midriff. Try

fabric that's gently gathered to flatter; face-framing necklines and heavier

styles draw attention up past the legs and tummy.

# ( 210 ) Appear thinner and taller with a ponytail

By changing how you wear your hair, you can create length, elongating your neck and face. Try this updated ponytail—it's perfect to take you from the beach to après-beach get-togethers. Just gently tease the crown of your hair using a comb, smooth the hair straight back with your hands without a part, and secure a high ponytail in the middle of your head. Loosen hair at the crown for a fuller look.

# ( 211 ) Workout clothes

If it's hot enough for the beach, chances are you're going to sweat like crazy when you work out. Wear looser clothing during your exercise routine, especially if you wear shorts or yoga pants. Built-up sweat can cause breakouts and heat rashes (not to mention yeast infections). And swear off spandex, which can trap sweat next to your skin.

## (212) Who wears short shorts?

• **To cover up your thighs,** look for shorts that resemble a flowing skirt. Or try loose-fitting shorts with an elastic waistband.

• **No butt?** Look for a pair of crazy-colored surfer shorts with a wild pattern.

• **If your legs are skinny,** wide-leg shorts make your legs look even skinnier. Go with short-shorts or even hot pants.

• **If you have short legs**, think short-shorts! The more showing, the better.

## (213) Did you know?

In the 1940s, the U.S. Department of Commerce measured body points on 10,000 American military women and assigned sizes between 2 and 20. Even though we still follow those guidelines, the average woman has changed from 5'2" and 129 pounds to 5'4" and 142 pounds.

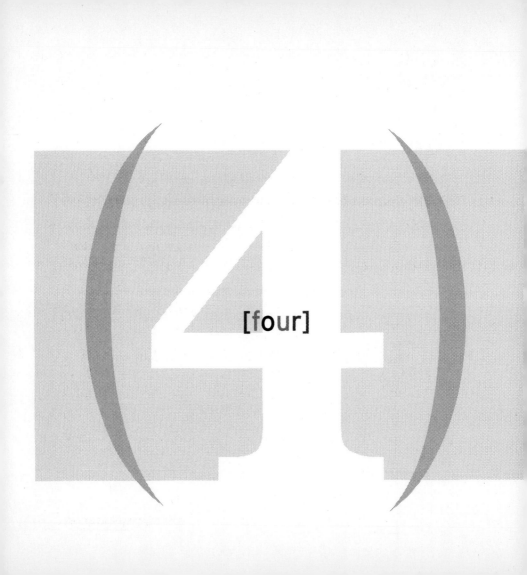

[four]

# The 9-to-5 Grind

**What do meetings, computers, and briefcases have** to do with great legs and butts? Everything! If you feel strong, healthy, and confident, a raise or promotion could be right on the other side of that boardroom door. Studies have even shown evidence that taller people receive more kudos at the office. So it's time to cause a little water cooler conversation. Even if you aren't 5'11", this chapter will teach you the right posture for confidence and height, how not to get sucked into the fast-food frenzy that is the corporate lunchroom, and how to work it at work when it comes to respect-commanding attire. And no one has to know that, underneath that pinstriped pantsuit, your legs and butt are to-die-for commodities in their own right. After all, how can you jump high enough to break that glass ceiling if you don't have strong legs for the boost? ~

## (214) Detox your legs

Pollution and other elements in the air can not only damage your skin, but they can also take away your healthy glow. Shine outside as well as inside by removing the toxins with a clay mask applied to your legs and backside. Try this simple at-home recipe:

Smooth a mixture of $^1/_2$ cup green or brown clay (available at health food stores) and $^1/_2$ cup plain yogurt over your body. Let it dry, then rinse with warm water.

# (215) Silky soft legs

Mix two tablespoons of petroleum jelly with the contents of one 400 IU Vitamin E capsule and massage all over your legs. Slip on cotton sweats and go to bed. In the morning, wash your legs with a moisturizing body wash and apply a body lotion. Your skin will be as soft as silk!

# (216) Speed healing with arnica

Have weekend activities like moving a friend or playing not-so-touch football left you with bruises that make your legs look like you're a professional stuntwoman? Rub on a cream or gel with at least 15 percent arnica oil. This essence from a daisylike flower stimulates white blood cells to fight bacteria around a bruise. Find these homeopathic lotions at health food stores and smooth some on bruised and battered legs.

## ( 217 ) Rub tired legs away

Rub your thighs with rosemary, peppermint, juniper, thyme oil—or any combination of these scents—for increased circulation and metabolism. Now you're ready to tackle the day.

## ( 218 ) How you sit can help fight cellulite

Sit on the edge of your office chair to stimulate lymphatic flow through the inner thigh glands and ducts. This will improve circulation and help aid in the fight against cellulite.

## ( **219** ) Exhilarate your legs with coffee grounds

A wake-up call for you and your skin! Take the cool coffee grounds
from your morning cup of coffee and rub them on your legs for a little
morning pick-me-up in the shower. The coffee exfoliates, and the aroma
is proven to elevate moods. And the grounds aren't as abrasive as some
salt-based scrubs.

## ( **220** ) Soothe razor burn

Wearing pantyhose all day can sometimes aggravate any razor burn
from shaving. Soothe the area with aloe vera or a cooling gel specifically
made for use after shaving. Avoid putting on heavy moisturizers that
might irritate or cause more problems, such as clogged pores.

# ( 221 ) Dry brushing

Use a dry brush to remove dead skin that dulls your otherwise glowing gams. Before your bath or shower, massage your dry legs and derriere using a circular motion with a bath brush. This method has been used for hundreds of years to remove dead skin cells from the body without removing the protective oils. Rinse away the dead cells, leaving touchable, softer skin.

# ( 222 ) Cover up with makeup

Your face isn't the only part of you that could benefit from a little cover-up. Hide bruises, birthmarks, and veins on your legs with body makeup. An opaque, natural finish will correct imperfections for a more beautiful body. Look for smudge-proof and water-resistant treatments that moisturize and protect the skin. Apply with your fingertips or a makeup sponge with smooth, even dabs and a blending motion. Let dry for 15 minutes before putting on clothing. Try stick or pot formulas or corrective foundation for large scars.

## (223) Your clothes could cause acne

If you have butt blemishes, avoid synthetic underwear. And if you wear thongs, remember that synthetic fibers in your clothes and hose can also cause these unsightly bumps. Keep it natural with cotton until the problem clears up.

## (224) Don't dry out

Can't live without a long, hot bath to soak away the day? To avoid drying out in the tub, coat your skin with oil before getting in. Just be careful not to slip!

# (225) The new hair removal

Sugaring involves applying a paste made primarily of sugar which is then removed from the skin (along with the hair) via a cloth strip. Unlike waxing, sugaring adheres only to your hair, not to your skin. Results usually last over a month. It costs around $60 for full-leg results.

### Egyptian Sugaring Paste

If you want to keep it cheap and sweet, try this at-home recipe:
• 2 cups sugar
• 1/4 cup lemon juice
• 1/4 cup water

Combine ingredients in a large saucepan. Stir constantly over low heat until the sugar is dark brown. Pour the mixture into a thick plastic storage container and allow it to cool until it's warm and spreadable. Test the temperature on a small portion of skin. If it has cooled too much, reheat it in the microwave for 10 to 20 seconds. Spread a thick layer of sugar on the desired area. Immediately cover with a cloth strip. Smooth down the cloth in the direction of hair growth. Hold one end of the strip taut as you pull the strip off in the opposite direction of hair growth.

## (226) Get the fitness fax

Work your calf muscles while faxing that important report. Put your hand against the fax machine to steady yourself and rest the top of your right foot on the back of your left. While waiting for your document to go through, lift up and down on your left leg. Do 10 reps, then switch legs.

## (227) Quick stair lifts for sculpted muscles

Stand at the bottom step of a set of stairs. Step up one foot at a time, placing your foot firmly in the center of the step. Bring the other foot up so both feet are on the step. Then step back down to the ground one foot at a time. This works your hamstrings, quads, calves, and butt.

# (228) How to sit to make more money

Studies report evidence that taller people can earn $790 a year more per inch over a lifetime, so sit tall! Good posture starts with your butt. Make sure that both cheeks are evenly on the chair. Your feet should both be on the floor or crossed at your ankles. Keep your pelvis neutral and make sure your shoulders are relaxed. Your chin should be parallel to the floor or tilted slightly down.

# (229) A workout while you work

It is possible to have a ball at work. Editors at a certain health and fitness magazine have even abandoned their desk chairs for stability balls. Sitting on the ball encourages good posture and trying to avoid falling off in front of co-workers means that you are constantly engaging your legs, glutes, and abs to keep your balance.

# (230) Create some resistance

Buy elastic resistance bands or stretch tubes for working different leg muscles. Different colored bands offer different levels of resistance. By pulling against a band anchored in a doorjamb or under your foot, you can challenge your hamstrings, quads, and glutes.

# (231) Go backwards

It may look ridiculous, but walking backwards on the treadmill or pedaling backwards on the elliptical trainer will excercise different muscles (especially the quads) than the usual forward motion does. But don't go too fast, because a wipeout will look even sillier in reverse.

# workbook

## ( 232 ) A quick leg workout

This workout targets all the muscles of your lower half and will guarantee a firm, round bottom and shapely legs in no time.

**CURTSY LUNGE WITH LEG LIFT** (works quads, hamstrings, buttocks, upper hips, and calves)

Stand with your feet slightly apart, legs straight, hands on hips (or holding a 5- to 8-pound dumbbell on each shoulder). Keeping your torso erect and your abs contracted, step back with your left foot, placing it behind your right foot, so the ball of your left foot is on the floor, heel lifted. Immediately bend both knees, keeping your torso straight and your front knee aligned with your front foot and back knee approaching floor. Push off your left foot, straightening your left leg and lifting it up and out to the side. Lower your left leg to starting position to finish reps, then switch legs to complete the set. Do one or two sets of 10 to 15 reps on each side.

**FRONT-TO-BACK TOE TOUCH** (works quads, hamstrings, buttocks, inner thighs, and upper hips)

Stand with your hands on your hips and your feet hip-width apart. Bend your left knee and extend your right leg in front of you, reaching as far forward with your toe as you can to touch the floor. Extend your right arm alongside your head and up into the air. Keeping your left knee bent, lift your right toe off the floor and bend your right knee, then shift your torso forward slightly from your hips as you swing your right leg back and extend it behind you.

Touch your right toe to the floor as you reach your arm out to the side.

Continue to alternate front and back touches for 12 to 15 reps, then switch sides. Do two sets on each side.

**SIDESTROKE SCISSORS** (works quads, hamstrings, buttocks, upper hips, and inner thighs)

Lie on your left side with your head supported on your upper arm, right palm on the floor in front of your shoulder. Bend both knees to about 90 degrees. Contract your abs so your hips are square. Extend your bottom leg forward and top leg back without rolling forward or backward. Bend both legs back to starting position and switch, extending your top leg forward and bottom leg back. Do two sets of 12 to 15 reps on each leg.

**FROGGY EXTENSION** (works buttocks and hamstrings)

Lie facedown on the floor with your knees bent at 90 degrees and slightly less than hip-width apart, feet flexed and heels together, with your toes turned out. Cross your forearms, placing your forehead on them. Contract your abs. Using your butt muscles, lift your thighs off the floor and pulse twice. Keeping your thighs lifted and butt contracted, separate your heels and extend your legs until they're almost straight. Bend your knees back to starting position, lower your thighs, and repeat. Do one set of 10 to 12 reps.

**TREE SQUAT** (works quads, hamstrings, buttocks, and calves)

Stand with your left foot flat against the inside of your right leg, left knee turned out. Place your hands together at your breastbone, or rest a 5- to 8-pound dumbbell on each shoulder. Contract your abs, keeping your shoulder blades down and back. Maintain this position, then bend your standing knee into a quarter-squat without leaning forward. Pause for two seconds; straighten your standing leg. Repeat for 8 to 12 reps, holding the squat position on the last rep for 20 to 30 seconds. Do one or two sets of 8 to 12 reps on each leg.

# (233) Throw away the scale

If you think you are going to be obsessive about it, toss this nemesis of your weight-loss plan in the trash. You should only weigh yourself once a week, and always at the same time (the best time is in the morning). Also, don't freak out about the numbers (muscle weighs more than fat, remember). Instead, measure by how your clothes are fitting around your hips, thighs, and butt.

# (234) Add hustle to your muscle

Kicking up your workout intensity a couple of times a week builds muscle, burns more calories, boosts your metabolism, and may just get you to greater gams quicker. So if you're walking, try jogging once a week. If you swim only a few laps, double it.

## ( 235 ) Check in with your personal trainer (between conference calls)

You may miss out on someone yelling, "You can do it!," but online personal training can save money and time, overcome problems getting to the gym, and encourage you to stay active. Many of these programs offer tips on incorporating fitness into your busy schedule and one-on-one fitness consultations with certified fitness professionals.

## ( 236 ) Avoid the vending machine

To avoid the inevitable afternoon trip to the vending machine for a sugary energy snack, try some isometric leg exercises to increase oxygen flow in the blood and help wake up the brain. Press your knees and outer thighs against the sides of your desk (if your desk is rather large, you may need to do this one leg at a time). Hold for 30 seconds and release. Repeat as needed.

# ( 237 ) Bike to work

Why sit in a car when you are going to sit at your desk all day? If it's possible, bike to work. Just 10 minutes of riding burns 80 calories. It's a great quad workout—all before your first morning meeting.

# ( 238 ) Take fido for a walk

Combine a leg workout with a little quality pooch time. After the 9-to-5 rat race, let both of you stretch your legs with a nice long walk. My dog Dazey is not only happy to see me, but she knows that the end of my day means the beginning of her fun. Most vets recommend two 20-minute walks a day; you'll burn around 85 calories each stroll.

# (239) Desk yoga

Take a few minutes out of your day for a little desk yoga. This routine will wake you and your muscles up.

- **Stand, place one foot on your desk,** with your extended leg straight and a slight bend in your supporting leg. Make a big circle over your head with your arms, hands together. Reach out toward your toes, twist at your torso and reverse the motion. This movement should be slow, controlled, and graceful.

- **Sit in your chair** and go limp like a rag doll. Be sure that your head is down to get the full stretch in your back. Hold this pose for 30 to 60 seconds.

- **Sitting in your chair, clasp your hands together,** intertwining your fingers with your palms facing you. Twist your wrists so that your palms now face away and bring your hands toward the ceiling, stretching your arms above your head. Try to squeeze your ears with your arms, as your hands reach toward the ceiling. Hold for three seconds, then release. Repeat three to five times.

# (240) Lunchtime isn't just for lunch

Get the most out of your lunch break by having a small snack and spending the rest of your time walking, running errands, or shopping. Thirty minutes of brisk walking will burn off 125 calories, and the fresh air will do you good.

# (241) Take the stairs

This certainly burns more calories than pushing the button for the elevator. Call it a foot-operated cardio machine. A 135-pound woman burns 8 calories per minute walking up stairs. Weigh more? Burn more! Whether you walk, jog, or run up or down the stairs, it really zeroes in on the butt and calves.

## (242) Reach for the sky

Instead of hitting your snooze button in the A.M., lay on your back across your bed, with your feet and arms dangling over the sides. Stretch your arms and legs so that it feels like you're trying to touch the ends of the room. Don't hold your breath, but hold the position for 15 seconds, then relax. When you stand up you'll be a leaner, more limber you.

## (243) A great at-your-desk thigh toner

Sit up straight with both feet flat on the floor. Inhale and lift your right thigh a few inches off the seat as you press your left foot into the floor. Hold for five deep breaths. Breathing normally, rotate your ankle five times to the right. Repeat, rotating to the left. Place your foot back on the floor. Repeat with your left leg.

## ( 244 ) Jump to it

Celebrate reaching your professional (or fitness) goals by jumping for joy. One recent British study showed that jumping up and down 50 times a day for six months increased bone density by nearly 3 percent. Not to mention the great calf muscle workout you'll get.

## ( 245 ) Late-afternoon delight

Save the morning for the bed, not the gym. Your body temperature, muscle strength, and VO2 max (a measure of how much oxygen your cardiovascular system can deliver to your muscles) peak between 4 P.M. and 8 P.M. Come early evening, you will have more stamina and flexibility and will be less injury prone.

# ( 246 ) Important news

Swollen legs might be a sign of a medical condition, including liver or kidney disorders, blood clots, or congestive heart failure. If you notice edema (the swelling of legs due to a buildup of fluid and heavy water retention) in either or both of your legs, contact your doctor immediately.

# ( 247 ) Instant relief

If your legs feel swollen and heavy, try these tricks for quick relief:

**Elevate your legs.** Swelling goes down faster when your feet are 6 to 12 inches higher than your heart. Raise your legs at night and at least several times day.

**Walk.** Inactivity can make your circulation sluggish. Muscle contractions help push your blood through your veins and back to your heart, keeping it from pooling in your legs.

# workbook

## Belly dancing beauties

The supple rolling motion of the abs, the undulating arms, and the staccato hip drops lure you out of your power suit and into the flowing sexy scarves of the belly dancer's world. This new aerobic craze works your legs, glutes, and abs, and raises your heart rate (along with that of anyone who sees you). Combine the following moves for an at-home trip to an exotic world. If the music you choose is sultry and slow, use snake arms, undulations, hip slides, and circles. If it's more energetic, do hip lifts and drops, traveling camel steps, and shimmies. For more belly dancing, see if your local gym offers classes or check out Rania Androniki Bossonis's book *Bellydancing for Fitness* (Fair Winds Press, 2004) and her series of workout DVDs and videos.

**Begin in the basic belly dancing position:** One leg extended forward like you were taking a step, weight on your back leg, back knee slightly bent, chest held high, stomach in, and arms rounded, held up and out in front of your chest. Then use the following moves to dance your way to a better body.

# (248) Ab roll

Contract the diaphragm and then the lower abs. Then you push the diaphragm out and then the lower ab. When you can control it, smooth it out to a roll.

# (249) Hip circles

Stand with your feet slightly more than hip-width apart, push your hips way out to the right and then bring them around back, to the left, then back to center. The movement is similar to spinning a hula hoop, but make the moves slower and lower. Keep your pelvis pivoting on an axis in a continuous circular movement.

# ( 250 ) Shimmy

Stand with your knees slightly bent and your feet together with your pelvis tucked under. Straighten your right leg. Next straighten your left leg while bending your right. The movement comes from the thighs. Once you have the movement down, create a quick constant vibration from the knees to the thighs. This is great for getting rid of cellulite.

# ( 251 ) Horizontal figure eight

With your knees bent and your feet hip-width apart, move your hips to create a fluid figure eight—front and to the right, back, up through the center across to the left front, back, then up through center.

# $\left(252\right)$ Hip lift

The goal of this move is to lift your hip up while the rest of your body

remains still, so isolation is important. Start with both knees slightly bent.

In the basic belly dancing position, lean back and keep your back straight.

Drop your hip down and lift it up on the beat.

# $\left(253\right)$ Hip accents

Push your hips outward to the sides with small, sudden thrusting movements.

## (254) Top taps

Stepping to the right, tap the ground with your left toe. Sweep your right arm outward to the side and raise your left arm over your left ear and sway to the right. Now step to the left one step and tap your right toe. Move your left arm outward and raise your right arm.

## (255) Camel walk

Put your left foot in front, with your right foot behind. Your left foot moves forward while your pelvis is pushed forward, then your right foot catches up with it. The moves should be on the balls of the feet. Repeat as you slowly move across the floor.

# ( 256 ) Get a massage

Not only will it relax and refresh you before you tackle your inbox, but it will also benefit your body by releasing toxins and lactic acid buildup, the culprits of leg cramping and muscle tightness. And consider your nervous system balanced—whether it needed soothing or stimulation. Try Shiatsu, an Oriental-based system of finger-pressure that treats special points along acupuncture "meridians" or the channels of energy flow in the body.

# ( 257 ) Quick kickboxing workout

For a workout anywhere, try this 15-minute cardio blast of kick-boxing with no rest in between movements. The lunge and kick movements work your glutes and legs. Be sure to end with a few minutes of good stretches.

**3 minutes:** Bend at the knees, while keeping your body vertical. While remaining in this stance, punch across your chest with your right arm to the left, then your left arm to the right, twisting at the waist.

**4 minutes:** Lift your right knee eight times, tapping your toe on the ground in front of you. Then your left knee eight times. All the while, make your arms simulate the constant rolling punches of a hanging punching bag in the air.

**4 minutes:** Kick your right leg out in front of you, then return it to center standing, then lunge back on your left leg. Switch legs. Punch forward with the opposite arm each time you lunge back.

**4 minutes:** Kick out to the side with your right leg as high as is comfortable. Bring your leg back to the center, as you cross jab your left arm to the right in front of you. Do this eight times, then switch legs.

# ( **258** ) The most important meal

If you are tempted to run out of the house without at least a little something to nosh on, drop the briefcase and car keys, and take a seat. In a recent study published in the *American Journal of Epidemiology,* researchers found that those who missed breakfast were 4.5 times more likely to be obese than breakfast eaters.

# ( **259** ) Grilled to low-fat perfection

Avoid hidden fat and calories the easy way by asking for your chicken, fish, or beef grilled. This means there probably won't be any high-fat butter, oil, or sauces used in the preparation. Teriyaki (although high in sodium), blackened, and Cajun options are also tasty and healthy.

# ( 260 ) Fast-food fixers

The "Fast Food Powers that Be" have finally begun addressing America's obesity problem with more low-cal options. If you have to go fast food (which, according to a Gallup poll, 57 percent of women ages 18 to 49 do once a week), choose a salad or grilled chicken sandwich to lighten the caloric load on your behind.

# ( 261 ) Keep frozen veggies on hand

Frozen vegetables are easy, quick, and rich in nutrients. Take them to work for a quick lunch you can heat in the microwave. Just add a few tablespoons of water at the bottom of the container for a steamed veggie treat. Season with black pepper, herbs, lemon juice, or a balsamic vinegar dressing.

## ( **262** ) Stay away from soda machines

Limit your caffeine intake. Caffeine acts as a diuretic, sucking water from your body and dehydrating your skin. This can lead to sallow skin and lost elasticity—not to mention what the hidden calories in soda will do to your derriere. If it's the fizz you crave, try a flavored sparkling water.

## ( **263** ) Think zinc

The trace mineral zinc assists in the maintenance of collagen and elastin fibers that give skin its firmness, helping to prevent sagging (meaning you'll have firmer leg tissue). It also links amino acids that are needed for the formation of collagen, essential in wound healing. You can find it in seafood, turkey, pork, soybeans, and mushrooms.

## ( **264** ) An apple a day

Stave off the munchies by crunching on an apple a day. These orbs of goodness have 5 grams of dietary fiber each. That's 20 percent of the recommended daily intake, all for the low price of only 80 calories. And the fiber will make you feel more full, so you will avoid snacking at your desk. Nothing fits better in your purse for an on-the-go treat.

## ( **265** ) High-fiber cereal

Check the label for at least 3 grams per serving, or stick with three sure things: oatmeal, Cheerios, or Kashi brand cereal. These are good sources of soluble fiber for a morning meal that will keep you full until lunchtime. If you add soy milk, there's a bonus: Studies show that eating 25 to 50 grams of soy protein a day can reduce harmful LDL cholesterol.

## ( **266** ) Avoid carbs after lunch

Don't overconsume starchy carbs, sugars, and fats that will bulk you up. Stay away from the pasta and potatoes as the day wears on, or all of those carbs will wear you out.

## ( **267** ) Take a drink

What happened on *The Sopranos?* Did you see who got voted off the island? Get involved with water-cooler gossip for more than just the latest dirt on your favorite shows. Your body needs at least 64 ounces of water a day. Keep a bottle at your desk and fill it throughout the day, or get off that fabulous fanny and walk over to the office fridge for a cold, filtered glass.

# (268) Have a coffee break

If you drink coffee, try it with skim milk. It's a great source of calcium and doesn't pack as many calories as the cream in a calorie-laden latte. And studies have shown that sipping coffee 30 minutes before a meal suppresses appetite by 35 percent and can even boost your metabolism by up to 5 percent.

# (269) Brown bag it

Bring your own lunch. This will keep you away from the fast food typically eaten by on-the-go business lunchers and stop you from grabbing a huge burger and fries from the office cafeteria. You can also control your portions and ingredients when you make lunch at home, meaning you won't end up eating a bunch of high-calorie foods you may not have even wanted.

# ( 270 ) Lunch meat madness

Stick to low- or non-fat turkey breast, chicken breast, or roast beef, and avoid bologna, salami, and other processed meats. They're high in fat and have a lot of water-retaining sodium in them. And stay away from the mayo; try spicy mustard if you want a tangy taste. Add a slice of tomato and lettuce for veggie benefits, and you've got a healthy lunch.

# ( 271 ) Lettuce on the outside?

Try layering lunch meat and cheese slices between thick, flat bunches of iceberg lettuce. It gives you a crunch, without the added carbs and calories of bread.

## (272) **Steam your clothes**

Wrinkles can make a garment look like it's puckering and pulling in the wrong places. Make sure your clothes are well pressed and that pleats sit flat. This will minimize your hips and make your butt look smaller.

## (273) **Blazers and suit coats**

Leave your blazer, suit coat, or cardigan unbuttoned to create maximum slimming vertical body lines.

# ( 274 ) Feminine in a corporate world: the pantsuit

Dressing in all one color is a sure-fire flatterer, so a pantsuit is a perfect option. Pin-stripes create length and thinning silhouettes. Choose longer jackets to hide larger bottoms and add a feminine cami or blouse to soften the look and draw attention to the face.

# ( 275 ) Long cardigan

The best long sweaters are in slimming, lightweight fabrics. Shorter lengths (from hip-length to right around the knee) look fresh and aren't as cumbersome as floor-length dusters. Wearing these are a great way to add vertical lines and hide your hips and tush.

# ( 276 ) Did you know?

During WWII, when there was a shortage of stockings, many women shaved their legs and used leg makeup to give the appearance of stockings.

# ( 277 ) Show a little support

If you know you will be on your feet all day at a presentation or because that's just what your job entails, wear support hose. Put them on before you get out of bed in the morning so your legs don't have a chance to swell. And since you're going to want to get the most wear possible out of your stockings, keep them in the freezer. It will make them more durable and less run-prone.

# workbook

## ( **278** ) Skirt the issue

If you want to hide your lower half, wear a skirt or dress instead of pants, which can draw attention to your thighs and butt. To showcase the best of your legs, opt for a skirt that falls at the most flattering point. Follow these tips to choose the most flattering skirts for you.

• **If you have short legs,** wear a mini and shoes with a low heel. To make a miniskirt more serious than playful for the office, add a tailored jacket, dark tights, and boots.

• **If you wish to add length,** avoid mid-calf or low-waist skirts. Long skirts can be worn with high heels for instant height, or choose pencil or A-line skirts that fall at or just below the knee and wear them with heels. Pair your skirt with a tailored top and you'll have a long, lean look.

- **If you are shapely,** try a skirt that hits just below the knees in an A-line or tailored cut. But avoid anything flowing (like lace or ruffles) below the knee; it will bring attention to the butt and hips.
- **If you have large calves and ankles,** wear long skirts.
- **To make thin legs more womanly,** choose a mid-calf skirt with a hem that stops at the shapeliest part of your legs.

# ( 279 ) Hosiery choices

What you wear on your legs can really define how your legs look. Here are a few tips to make sure that you choose the most flattering hosiery:

- **Panty hose colors** should tie an outfit together, not be the outfit's focus. And stay away from bright colors, which can also add pounds.
- **For a thinning, monochromatic look,** choose dark, neutral hosiery such as charcoal, navy, or black with a dark bottom and shoes.

- **Although bare looks sexy,** it's not exactly professional, so choose nude (an exact skin-tone match) hose for that popular bare-legged look in casual situations.
- **To hide heavy legs,** choose thin tights to minimize leg size. Thick opaque tights on larger legs can make them look like masses of color.
- **Avoid high contrast** between your hosiery and shoe colors (such as white hose with black shoes).
- **One simple rule:** Never wear white hosiery unless you are a nurse or a bride.
- **The sheerer the hose,** the dressier the look. Choose semi-sheer for day, sheer for evening.
- **For a little butt shaping,** try figure-enhancing hosiery that creates a smooth, firming shape that lifts and shapes the wearer's bottom.

# ( 280 ) Not your granny's girdle

Don't underestimate the power of girdles and body-slimming shapers. They are much more comfortable than in days of old, but they have the same amazing power to get you into a fitted and unforgiving outfit.

# ( 281 ) Go off the cuff

If you have shorter legs, avoid wearing cuffed pants. Cuffed trousers can overpower the legs and break up the long lines of your body.

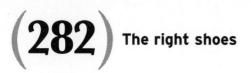

## The right shoes

Keep heels to $1\frac{1}{2}$ inches in the office. And stay away from chunky heels, which will make you look foot-heavy and draw attention to any ankle thickness. A feminine round toe has a "Minnie Mouse" effect that makes the foot look smaller, while super pointy shoes look awkward with a rounded butt and thicker legs.

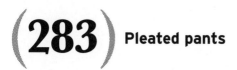

## Pleated pants

These are classic masculine pants, so they usually have a larger leg cut, which is perfect for hiding larger thighs. Be careful with fit, though. Pleated pants can also add weight to the hip area if they are not properly fitted.

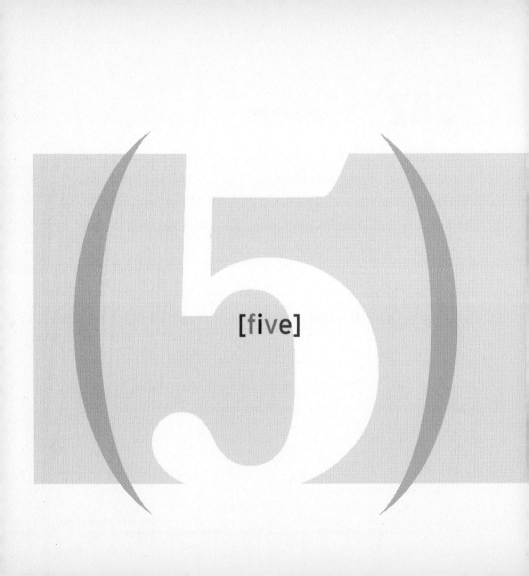

[five]

# Party Plans

**We've all had this nightmare before: You're staring** blankly at your open closet. It seems like your shoes are sticking their tongues out at you; your turtlenecks are hiding their heads in shame. It's the night of "the" party. Everyone you want to impress will be there, plus a few people you haven't even thought of yet. The problem is, the only thing "impressing" right now is the idea there is not an outfit in sight. There are things to wear, but you have nothing to Wear.

A wedding reception or a birthday bash, a reunion or just a get-together for cocktails—no matter what the reason to celebrate, make an entrance to a great party looking great, from top to fantastic bottom. And before you don that amazing ensemble, take a few moments to try out these exercise and beauty tips that will pull your look together. You'll be the "someone" that "everyone" will be talking about the next day. ~

*Health and Beauty Bytes*

# ( 284 ) Wrap it up

Body wraps can sometimes diminish cellulite and cause thigh inches to melt away (even if it's just for a few hours). If your neighborhood spa is booked, try this at-home wrap:

**Turn up the heat in your bathroom or bedroom.** Combine 8 drops of grapefruit essential oil; 2 drops each of thyme, fennel, lavender, geranium, and juniper berry essential oils; and 2 cups of almond oil. Shake well. Exfoliate your skin with a loofah, and spritz your body with the oil. Knead it into your legs and glutes, then wrap those areas snugly in plastic wrap. Relax in a warm room for 20 minutes, then remove the plastic. Shower with warm water.

## ( 285 ) Kicks butts for a nicer butt

Carbon monoxide can decrease your circulation and can contribute to cellulite. The list of reasons to quit just keeps getting longer.

## ( 286 ) Rub away cellulite

When our lymphatic system doesn't filter waste properly, toxic products accumulate and inflate the fat cells. Then it's Cellulite City. Encourage healthy lymph flow by massaging your legs and butt or by brushing them gently with a natural-bristle brush every morning before taking a shower. Always massage toward your heart, using circular motions.

# ( 287 ) Bath or shower?

Shower power! They are quicker, so your skin doesn't dry out. Use warm (not hot) water and a moisturizing soap or body wash. Voilà! You'll get clean skin and tons of time to get ready.

# ( 288 ) Dab on a slimming scent

Wear a floral and spice fragrance and you might appear slimmer. Researchers at the Smell and Taste Treatment and Research Foundation in Chicago had thousands of men inhale scents and then guess how much the women who wore them weighed. Women who wore spicy floral blends scored lower numbers; they were perceived to weigh an average of 12 pounds less than their actual weight.

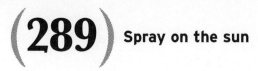

## ( 289 ) Spray on the sun

Create the illusion of shapely thighs and cut calves to show off in the shortest of party dresses. Some salons can "chisel" legs by spraying more tanning color in some places, less in others. The bronzed, subtly muscled look lasts about five days.

## ( 290 ) Pampered feet

Open-toe shoes call for a pedicure. It's the icing on the cake that is your lean and luxurious lower half. Don't want to spring for a salon job? Give yourself this simple home version:

1. Soak your feet in warm, soapy water.
2. Clip and file your nails straight across to avoid ingrown nails later.
3. Drop olive oil onto each toe and heel. Massage it in.
4. Finish with a coat of the prettiest of pinks or the raciest of reds.

# ( **291** ) Take care of your knees, please

You can't have great legs if your knees and ankles are cracked and dry. Smooth on the cocoa butter.

# ( **292** ) Picture perfect

When taking a photo, make sure your legs are the best-looking in the bunch with these tricks of the trade from model Suzanne Keck.
Say (fat-free jalapeño jack) cheese!

- **Never face your body straight toward the camera;** always stand at an angle.
- **Always extend the leg facing toward camera,** rather than tucking it behind your back leg, which visually cuts the lines of the body and makes you look heavier.
- **While sitting, never put your full weight on your thighs;** try to keep them at an angle, to one side or the other, and slightly lift

them off your chair. Flex your leg muscles to create definition, reduce the appearance of cellulite, and thin the overall appearance of your legs. If your legs are crossed for the photo, always slightly lift the top leg to produce the same effect.

- **Never cross your arms across your body.** This cuts the body up and makes each portion look larger. Also, your arms look larger when they are pushed against your body. Try to keep them in a flexed position to enhance muscles.
- **Keep your shoulders back,** breasts out, and back slightly arched to show the curve in your spine, waist, and buttocks.

## ( 293 ) Baby oil sexy shimmer

Smooth a thin layer of baby oil on your legs after bathing and while your skin is still a little moist. This seals moisture in, and it gives you a sexy glisten to your gams. Perfect for that flirty party mini.

# (294) Tattoos

Once seen only as a tribal ritual of far-off Egyptian tribes in the 1300s or the mark of a pierced and proud punk, even the most conservative of professionals now sport tattoos. They're a statement of individuality. According to the American Academy of Dermatology, the number of tattoo parlors has increased from 300 to more than 4,000 nationally in the past 20 years.

**GETTING INK DONE** A small needle injects ink into the dermal layer of the skin to create a permanent design. A small tattoo can take about 45 minutes, while larger ones can take much longer, even requiring repeat visits. If you choose to get tattooed and you aren't swayed by the risks (possible exposure to Hepatitis C and HIV, allergic reactions to the ink, and localized infection), obviously choose a reputable place. In most states these body art studios are not regulated by state health departments, so it's up to you to protect yourself by finding a salon that is clean and safe.

**Make sure:**

• The equipment is sterilized between each use.

• Needles are never reused. They should be unwrapped in front of you and thrown away after use.

• Inks are never reused.

• Gloves are used and replaced between procedures or after touching nonsterile items.

• References are available.

**HENNA TATTOOS** Want the whimsy of a tattoo but not the will-I-still-like-this-in-30-years staying power of one? Try the art of henna painting. Known as mendhi, this is safe, painless, and temporary, lasting anywhere from 2 to 12 weeks. Potent natural dye that ranges from an orange shade to a deep brick or red-brown is painted on the skin. You might have seen henna used for traditional body ornamentation on the palms and the soles of the feet during certain ceremonies of Middle Eastern and North African women.

## GETTING RID OF A TATTOO

Don't expect to have silky smooth, colorless skin when the tattoo removal process is completed. This isn't magic, it's medicine. In most cases, some scarring or color variations will remain, depending on the size and location. One of the following methods will be used to remove an existing tattoo.

**Excision.** Used especially when the tattoo is small. The advantage of this method is that the entire tattoo can be removed. After a local anesthetic, the entire design is removed surgically. The skin edges are brought together and sutured.

**Dermabrasion.** A small portion of the tattoo is sprayed with a solution that freezes the area. The tattoo is then "sanded" with a rotary abrasive instrument that causes the skin to peel.

**Laser.** Pulses of light from a laser are directed onto the tattoo, breaking up the color pigments. Over the next several weeks, the body's cells remove the treated pigmented areas. More than one treatment is usually necessary. This is one of the most recent popular methods.

**Salabrasion.** This is a centuries-old method; local anesthetic is used on and around the area after which a solution of salt water is applied. An abrading apparatus similar to the one used in dermabrasion is used to vigorously scrub the area. When the area becomes deep red in color, a dressing is applied.

# ( 295 ) Showgirl kicks

Show up those dancing darlings with your best showgirl kicks. Sit on the floor, knees bent, and legs together. Lean back so that your toes touch the floor, supporting your weight with your elbows behind you and palms flat. Drop your legs to the right, then left, and kick your legs up as high as you can. Draw your knees back to center and repeat to the left. Do 8 to 15 reps.

# ( 296 ) Get this party started

Turn on your radio and pump up the volume while you're picking out your outfit. Not only will this get you jazzed for a fun night out, but it will also burn about 75 calories in 10 minutes.

# ( 297 ) Mix it up

Believe it or not, your muscles have a memory. If you usually lift weights in a certain order, it's certain that your body will get bored. So change it up. Do leg lifts after squats one day, then switch it around for the next workout. It will shock your muscles into wondering what's next and make them work a little harder.

# ( 298 ) Pick up that microphone

Yes, it's cheesy, but it can help burn off the bleu from the hors d'oeuvres tray you were just hovering over. Belt out a song on a karaoke machine and you can sing goodbye to 20 calories. And once you have their attention, put in a few dance moves (think fame and glory for your gams!)

# ( **299** ) Upper-body workout

Fitness experts suggest that rather than focusing on your lower body alone, you should combine strength-training moves, like squats and lunges, with upper-body work (maybe a bicep curl or two?), which will bring your figure into balance. The sculpted and stronger upper body takes emphasis away from your thighs. When you're at the gym, do more press-ups, triceps dips, and shoulder presses.  And if you need more incentive, here's an added bonus: Each pound of muscle you gain from lifting weights increases your resting metabolic rate by about 30 to 40 calories per day.

# ( **300** ) You spin me right round

Spin your way to a fantastic fanny with a spinning class. These indoor biking classes really get you going, with pumping music and an instructor to get your butt in gear. After some warm-up exercises on the bike, tricks like standing up on the bike while pedaling whip your butt into shape (to the tune of more than 600 calories an hour). A resistance knob makes the ride more realistic, as you pump your legs up hills and down descents. Some classes even provide a screen with scenery. If your gym doesn't offer a spinning class, call 800-847-SPIN for programs in your area.

# (301) Relax!

Stress can cause increased storage of fat around the hips and abs. Add together years of worrying and you can actually disrupt your fat cells' ability to make estrogen, causing them to expand in an effort to compensate. Find ways to release your stress—journal writing, therapy, or talking to friends and family.

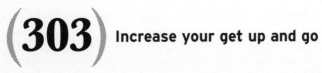

## (302) Increase your balance

Stand on one leg with your knee slightly bent and your arms tight against your sides. Balance on your leg for 10 to 30 seconds and then drop your weight a little and hold for 10 to 30 seconds more. Repeat this sequence three or four times with your knee bent to various degrees, and repeat with the other leg. To make it more challenging, do the same sequence with your eyes closed. This also works the quads and hamstrings.

## (303) Increase your get up and go

For more energy, lie on the floor with your heels up against a wall for 10 to 15 minutes. Now you're ready to get those legs movin'!

# ( 304 ) A change of pace

For great-looking legs, shake things up by walking backwards and sideways. It may look stupid, but this will wake up muscles and shape them fast. Because these are unnatural moves, try this routine on a track or treadmill. Go through this sequence twice for a 50-minute workout that will burn 340 calories.

| Time | Pace | Speed | Incline |
|------|------|-------|---------|
| 5 minutes | warm-up | 3.3-3.8 mph | 1-2% |
| 4 minutes | fast-forward | 4.5 mph | 1-2% |
| 1 minute | recovery | 4 mph | 1-2% |
| 4 minutes | backward steps | 1-1.5 mph | 0-2% |
| 1 minute | recovery | 4 mph | 1-2% |
| 4 minutes | uphill | 3.3-3.8 mph | 8-15% |
| 1 minute | recovery | 4 mph | 1-2% |
| 4 minutes | side-to-side shuffles | 1 mph | 1-2% |
| 1 minute | recovery | 4 mph | 1-2% |

## ( 305 ) Stand tall

Confidence gets you noticed. Saggy shoulders, slumped backs, and drooping butts don't. Check your posture by standing sideways in front of a mirror. Your ears, shoulders, and hips should be in alignment. Turn to face the mirror and let your arms hang naturally. If you can see the backs of your hands, your shoulders are rounded too far forward.

## ( 306 ) At the gym

Those big cardio machines may seem intimidating, but show them who's boss and you'll be rewarded with strong legs and glutes.

**Stationary exercise bikes.** Try the upright bike when you are looking to focus on your thighs and the recumbent version when you want to focus more on your butt.

**Rowing machines.** Your quads, abs, and upper body will benefit from this nautical workout.

**Stair steppers**. These longtime favorites place special emphasis on the butt and calves. For the best butt-blasting workout, use the rolling staircase version. For the workout that's easiest on the knees, try the recumbent version.

**Elliptical trainer.** Use this to add hills to your routine for additional leg sculpting.

**Treadmill.** Increase the incline of your walking or running workout to place more emphasis on your butt muscles. Alternate sprinting with walking to boost your metabolism.

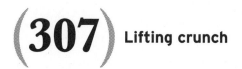 **Lifting crunch**

Lie on your back with your knees bent, feet slightly apart, and arms down at your sides. Squeeze your glutes together and tighten your abs. Continue to squeeze your butt as you raise your pelvis toward the ceiling, lifting as high as you can. Hold for three counts. Keeping your glutes tight, slowly lower your pelvis down to the floor, rolling down from the top vertebra to your tailbone.

# workbook

## ( 308 ) One-minute cardio moves

**Jumping jacks.** Stand with your feet together, then jump, separating your legs and raising your arms overhead. Land with your feet hip-width apart, then jump your feet back together and lower your arms.

**Stair running.** Run up a flight of stairs, pumping your arms, then walk down. Vary by taking two stairs at a time.

**Jumping rope.** Stay on the balls of your feet, not jumping too high off the ground and keep your elbows by your side.

**Squat jump.** Stand with feet hip-width apart, arms bent at your sides. Bend your knees and lower your hips into a squat. Jump in the air and straighten your legs to land, raising your arms straight into the air above your head. Return to the squat for your next jump, bringing your arms back down to your side.

**Split jump.** Stand in a split stance, one foot a long stride in front of the other, then bend your knees and jump, switching legs to land and pumping arms in opposition to legs. Alternate legs.

**Step-up.** Step up on a curb, stair, or sturdy bench with one foot, then the other, then down one at a time. Repeat.

**Alternating knee lift.** Stand tall and bring one knee toward your chest without collapsing your rib cage; twist your opposite elbow toward your raised knee. Alternate sides.

**Hamstring curl.** Stand tall and step sideways with your right foot, then bring your left heel toward your buttocks. Alternate sides, keeping your elbows pulled in close to your body.

**Jog in place.** Lift your knees up while swinging your arms naturally in opposition. Land softly, rolling from the balls of your feet to your heels.

**Side-to-side leap.** Place any long, thin object (such as a broom) on the floor. Leap sideways over the object, landing with feet together.

# ( **309** ) Classic Pilates moves for sleek leg lines

To begin: Lie on your side, abs pulled in, bottom arm stretched out under your head, and top arm placed in front of you for support. Stretch your body as straight and long as possible.

**Front and back kicks.** Lift your top leg about six inches, point your toes, and pulse the leg forward two times, then back two times. When pulsing back, be sure to squeeze your buttocks. Do 15 on each side.

**Up and down kicks.** Slightly turn out your top leg and lift it as high as you can without rolling back. Then slowly pull your leg back down in along line with muscles engaged. Do 15 on each side.

**Leg beats.** Lift your top leg about twelve inches and bring your bottom leg up to meet it. Slowly lower to the floor and do 15 times on each side.

**Leg circles.** Lay on your back with one leg pointed straight up into the air. Make 10 small clockwise circles, then switch direction, for a total of 20 circles with each leg.

# workbook

## ( 310 ) Lunges and squats

A lunge is the ultimate butt and leg workout. Always remember: Never lock your knees at the top, and never let your knees bend past your toes.

**THE LUNGE:** Step back from a standing position with one leg. Move down toward the floor by bending your front leg in a controlled manner until your back knee comes close to touching the floor. Push with your front leg while squeezing your butt to move back into the starting position. Try one full set of 10, then switch legs. Do three sets of 10.

**Variation:** The traveling lunge is a basic lunge, but instead of moving back into the starting position, you move forward into the next lunge.

**THE SUMO SQUAT:** Stand with your feet wider than shoulder width and your toes pointing out. Slowly bend both knees to squat as deeply as you can. Press up. Do three sets of 5 to 10 reps.

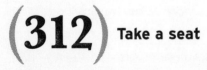

*Nutrition Nuggets*

# (311) Skip the cake frosting

When you're in charge of bringing the cake, skip the store-bought frosting in favor of your own fruity fat-free stuff. You can cut 1,155 calories and 48 grams of fat. Peel 6 medium, firm peaches and puree them in a food processor along with 2 teaspoons of apple juice and 1 tablespoon of sugar. Top your cake with this and you'll spread holiday cheer, not your hip-width.

# (312) Take a seat

Don't eat standing up. Make it a rule. If you have to sit down to eat, you'll eat more slowly and maybe less often.

# ( **313** ) Alternate alcohol with virgin drinks

Space out your party beverages—have a glass of sparkling water after a glass of wine or a mixed drink. Alcohol has calories galore and can make you nibble more (not to mention help you say bye-bye to your inhibitions!).

# ( **314** ) Choose a smaller plate

At a buffet party, ask your hostess for a smaller plate. That way you will be forced to take less food, rather than filling up your plate and creating a diet disaster. And keep this fact in mind as you cruise the holiday buffets: A study at Tufts University found that half of the average population's annual weight gain occurs during the last six weeks of the year. If you can behave for just a month and a half, you might make one fewer resolution this January!

# ( 315 ) Marinate for flavor, not fat

For a BBQ, give the main course more flavor by marinating it for 24 hours. Then you can forego the creamy sauces and fatty gravies. For chicken, try lemon zest and rosemary; give your salmon a sprinkle of cumin and a drizzle of olive oil.

# ( 316 ) Low-fat chips and dips

If you're throwing the party, use low- or non-fat chips. Choosing fat-free potato chips could save up to 300 calories per person. For dips, try salsa, which is fat-free, or use reduced-fat sour cream, very little mayonnaise, or nonfat yogurt. Use fresh herbs and spices (like parsley and cilantro) and hot pepper sauce to add great flavor.

## ( 317 ) Stop eating after 9 P.M.

An all-night party shouldn't mean an all-night food fest. Experts suggest you stop eating a few hours before bedtime. This will give you time to digest before your body rests. On a full stomach, not only will you not burn off the calories well, but you risk having a fitful night's sleep and potential leg cramps.

## ( 318 ) Halt the salt

Stay away from party foods like salty pretzels, peanuts, and chips. Too much sodium increases swelling and water retention, leaving you with bloated legs and ankles. Instead, grab a piece of cheese and some crackers to fill you up—or better yet, munch on fare from the veggie plate.

## (319) Sip cranberry juice

Drink spirits and they will come back to haunt you as body bloat. Combat this puffy problem by sipping a cranberry juice concoction of half water, half juice. This diuretic will flush out any salt that might keep your legs from looking and feeling their best.

## (320) Never show up hungry

To keep your cravings under wraps, never go to a party hungry. Have a snack before you hit the social circuit, so you aren't tempted with calorie-laden appetizers. This will give you more time to socialize and less need to nosh on hip-widening munchies. Try an apple, some yogurt, or even a bowl of cereal.

## (321) Beverage foes

In order to lose one pound of fat, which equals about 3,500 calories, you have to create a 500-calorie deficit each day of the week. So cut out soda and juice, which can have as much as 200 calories each glass. Drink water instead. Water also helps keep the skin plump and hydrated, which means less dimpling on the wrong cheeks.

## (322) Grab a handful of almonds

Snack on a handful of almonds as you run out the door. Full of calcium, fiber, and Vitamin E, these little gems will fill you up so that you don't find yourself gravitating toward the guacamole and chips during the party.

## (323) Weighty weekends

A study in *Obesity Research* reveals that we consume 115 calories more per day on Friday, Saturday, and Sunday, mostly from fat and alcohol. This adds up to six pounds a year. Break the pattern and try to stay on track, despite your social calendar.

## (324) Stave off leg cramps

Legs cramping up? The old wives' tale of eating a banana to make cramps go away is actually true. Potassium aids in muscle contractions, and a deficiency of potassium can cause cramping. In addition to bananas, you can find potassium in potatoes, strawberries, cantaloupes, tomatoes, and fruit juices. So dance the night away cramp-free!

## ( 325 ) Add fat for softer skin?

Forget fat-free diets. A lack of fat in your diet can cause your skin to become dry, and that means itchy legs. Stick to healthy, unsaturated fats (found in olive oil, fatty fish, and almonds) for smooth skin.

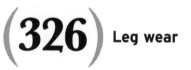

## ( 326 ) Leg wear

Spice up an outfit and draw attention to your great gams with textured panty hose or tights. Stay away from horizontal stripes, though, as they tend to make your legs seem bigger than they are. Thicker fabric tights are another inch-adding no-no.

# (327) Create length with a skirt slit

To make your legs (or at least one of them) look thinner, tempt your viewers with a sneaky peek through a slit in your skirt. The sight line will create length by drawing the eyes up and down. Pair a long skirt with a high slit with sexy fishnets or shimmery nylons.

# (328) Dress it up

Make an entrance in the perfectly selected party dress to show off your best assets. Follow these tips to avoid a dress disaster:

- Play down a pear shape with a full skirt.
- Enhance a boyish figure with gathered fabric, to enhance curves.
- Appear taller in a strapless mini dress.
- Create curves with feminine layers of chiffon and ruffles.
- Look leaner in a column dress.
- Minimize a big butt with an slightly flared A-line skirt.

# ( 329 ) Coverage hosiery

The bare-legged look may seem chic, but it's not when there you have varicose veins, uneven tans, and razor stubble to contend with. Not to mention the lack of a control top. Instead, opt for nude-colored, sheer panty hose (sandalfoot, of course) to get the same look plus an elegant smoothness.

# ( 330 ) Party coats

- **If you're curvy,** find a straight, sleek style that nips in where your waist does and hits at the knee.
- **If you're skinny,** add a little curve to your body with a quilted coat.
- **If you're tall,** opt for a knee-length or mid-calf coat that's tailored slightly at the waist.
- **If you're petite,** hit-the-hip styles make legs look inches taller. Make sure the shoulders are a narrow, not wide fit.

# (331) To hide 5 pounds:

Perform a quick butt-and-thigh disappearing act with a body slimmer or shaper. Try a body slip to give yourself a sexy silhouette under today's body-hugging looks, or a bodysuit with side panels to hold in saddlebags and contour your rear. Use a bottom booster to make pancake ass a thing of the past, and slip into a stomach-to-hip-and-thigh slimmer before you zip up a tight pencil skirt. If you need a sleek look from head to toe, try a ribcage to thigh support with waist paneling. And if you need just a bit of extra help under miniskirts, count on Lycra-fortified boy shorts to minimize bulges around the stomach and lift the butt. Tips for choosing the perfect body shaper:

- **Check for the Lycra level**—it's the squeezing power. The lightest control is less than 15 percent, the firmest has 35 percent or more.
- **Shapers should be so tight** that they are hard to pull on. Once in place, they should feel comfortable. You should be able to slip two fingers into the waistband.

- **Try the shaper** on with what you plan on wearing it under.
- **Stand in natural light** to make sure the slimmer doesn't show through your clothes.

# (**332**) Fur trims

Call everyone's attention to your best feature—your face—with faux fur trim collars. This glam flattery trick will make you feel confident and look like a diva! All the while you'll be bringing their eyes up, not down.

# (**333**) Leave the trends for the teens

Wear your clothes; don't let them wear you. Limit trendy pieces so you will have more wardrobe flexibility. And nothing tells the world you are standing on two strong legs more than classic style and elegance do.

# ( **334** ) Shiny happy bodies

Caution: Objects may appear larger in shiny fabric. Avoid reflective fabric (especially in the butt and hip areas) that draws attention.

# ( **335** ) Ways to wear a mini

- **Fake a tan:** This makes legs look longer and thinner.
- **Wear nude tights:** Add a bit of shine with Lycra.
- **Reel in some attention with fishnets:** A little bit sexy, yet still fashion-conscious. Flesh-tone fishnets are fashion's best-kept secret.
- **Pay attention to proportion:** An off-the-shoulder top or gathered neckline balances the smallness of the skirt below.
- **Slip on some great shoes:** Try sexy pointed flat shoes with miniskirts.
- **Regress a little:** For a younger look, try a tall boot with a flat heel.

## ( 336 ) Thinner fabric means a thinner you

Thinner fabric will give your body a slim and willowy appearance.
Heavy wool and winter fabrics tend to add about a $^1/_4$ inch to your body.

## ( 337 ) Choosing your shoes

- **Wear heels**—even a $1^1/_2$-inch heel extends the line of the leg.
- **Choose tapered toes** with low vamps—the more foot you show, the longer your legs appear.
- **Stacked heels, slingbacks, and elongated mules** lengthen your legs by anchoring your heels and creating weight at the bottom of your feet. (This distracts from your legs' width.)
- **If you have a short body,** avoid spiky stilettos.
- **Beware of shoes with ankle straps and T-straps;** they can cut legs off at the ankle, adding extra pounds.
- **Pump up the color** to draw attention to a great set of ankles and legs.

# [acknowledgments & sources]

I would like to thank the following for their assistance in my
information gathering:

American Center for Dermatology
American Council on Exercise
American Dietetic Association
American Journal of Epidemiology
Calorie Control Council
Centers for Disease Control
Corinne Cafferky, licensed aesthetician, Boston
IDEA: The Health & Fitness Source
Elyse Jacob, Kartel Kollections, Los Angeles
Suzanne Keck
Samantha Slaven, Samantha Slaven Publicity,
Los Angeles Florence Tambone
www.Dermadoctor.com
www.healthatoz.com

# [about the author]

**Cheryl Fenton** is a Boston-based freelance writer who has been in the
magazine industry for thirteen years, with bylines in *Women's Health and Fitness*,
*Walking* and *InStyle*. She is a regular at the gym and a big fan of lunges, with 43
pairs of tall boots and high-heeled strappy sandals to wear with the shortest of
minis for showing off her results.